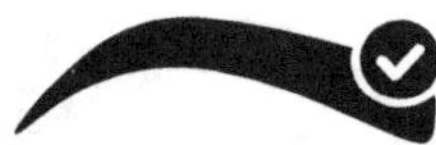

Healing process after micropigmentation

The healing process following permanent eyebrow makeup takes place in several stages and usually lasts between 4 to 6 weeks. During this time, the appearance of your eyebrows will change as the pigment gradually settles into the skin. Below are the stages of the healing process:

1. **Day 1: Immediately After the Procedure**
   Your eyebrows will look very intense, dark, and prominent. The skin may be slightly swollen and red. The pigment will appear darker than the final result, as the dye is still on the surface of the skin.

2. **Days 2–3**
   Swelling starts to subside, and the skin around the eyebrows may feel dry or tight.
   The eyebrows will still appear dark, but the skin begins to form a light protective layer.

3. **Days 4–7**
   Exfoliation begins. Scabs may form and fall off naturally, so it's important not to touch, scratch, or try to speed up the process.
   Your eyebrows may look uneven or have „empty" spots, but this is a normal part of healing as the pigment settles.

4. **Days 7–14**
   The scabs gradually fall off, and the pigment may look much lighter. Many people feel that their eyebrows are too light at this stage, but the color will continue to stabilize.
   Continue to avoid excessive washing and using cosmetics on the eyebrow area.

5. **Days 14–21**
   The eyebrows will appear lighter and more natural. Some areas may seem lighter than others, but this is part of the process.
   The pigment begins to settle into the skin, and the final color will start to become more visible.

6. **After 4 Weeks**
   By this point, the eyebrows are fully healed. The color will be 20-50% lighter compared to the first few days post-procedure.
   A touch-up session may be needed to fill any pigment gaps or refine the shape.

Date of your touch-up:

Post-procedure care after micropigmentation

Following a micropigmentation procedure, the skin requires special attention to ensure proper healing and long-lasting, aesthetic results. Below are the recommended post-care instructions:

1. **Hygiene**

   Always wash your hands before touching your eyebrows.

   For the first week, gently cleanse the treated area with lukewarm water.

   Soak a cotton pad in lukewarm water and gently dab your eyebrows, avoiding any rubbing motions.

   Dry the area using a dry cotton pad, again with gentle dabbing to avoid friction.

   Repeat this process 4 times a day at regular intervals.

   For the first two weeks, avoid excessive moisture on the eyebrows (e.g., during baths or showers). After 7-14 days, when the initial healing has occurred, you may begin using a gentle micellar water for cleansing. Avoid products containing alcohol or harsh ingredients.

2. **Preventing Irritation**

   Do not scratch or rub your eyebrows, even if small scabs form. Allow the scabs to fall off naturally to avoid scarring or pigment loss.

   Avoid applying makeup to the eyebrow area until fully healed (approximately 7-14 days).

   For at least 14 days, avoid saunas, swimming pools, hot baths, and excessive sweating, as these can cause the pigment to fade or irritate the skin.

3. **Sun Protection**

   Avoid sun exposure and tanning beds for at least 4 weeks. UV radiation can cause the pigment to fade.

   Once your eyebrows are fully healed, apply a high SPF sunscreen to protect the pigment from fading.

4. **Avoiding Intensive Cosmetic Treatments**

   For 4-6 weeks post-procedure, avoid facial treatments such as chemical peels, laser treatments, or the use of strong creams around the eyebrow area, as these may weaken the pigment.

5. **Consulting a Specialist**

   If you have any concerns or notice unusual symptoms such as excessive redness, swelling, or oozing, contact the cosmetologist who performed the procedure.

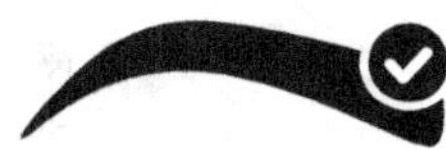

Healing process after micropigmentation

The healing process following permanent eyebrow makeup takes place in several stages and usually lasts between 4 to 6 weeks. During this time, the appearance of your eyebrows will change as the pigment gradually settles into the skin. Below are the stages of the healing process:

(1) **Day 1: Immediately After the Procedure**

Your eyebrows will look very intense, dark, and prominent. The skin may be slightly swollen and red. The pigment will appear darker than the final result, as the dye is still on the surface of the skin.

(2) **Days 2–3**

Swelling starts to subside, and the skin around the eyebrows may feel dry or tight.
The eyebrows will still appear dark, but the skin begins to form a light protective layer.

(3) **Days 4–7**

Exfoliation begins. Scabs may form and fall off naturally, so it's important not to touch, scratch, or try to speed up the process.
Your eyebrows may look uneven or have „empty" spots, but this is a normal part of healing as the pigment settles.

(4) **Days 7–14**

The scabs gradually fall off, and the pigment may look much lighter. Many people feel that their eyebrows are too light at this stage, but the color will continue to stabilize.
Continue to avoid excessive washing and using cosmetics on the eyebrow area.

(5) **Days 14–21**

The eyebrows will appear lighter and more natural. Some areas may seem lighter than others, but this is part of the process.
The pigment begins to settle into the skin, and the final color will start to become more visible.

(6) **After 4 Weeks**

By this point, the eyebrows are fully healed. The color will be 20-50% lighter compared to the first few days post-procedure.
A touch-up session may be needed to fill any pigment gaps or refine the shape.

Date of your touch-up:

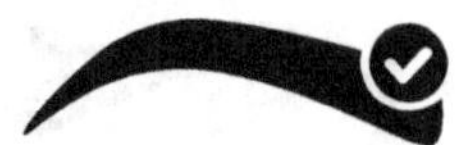

Post-procedure care after micropigmentation

Following a micropigmentation procedure, the skin requires special attention to ensure proper healing and long-lasting, aesthetic results. Below are the recommended post-care instructions:

1. **Hygiene**

   Always wash your hands before touching your eyebrows.

   For the first week, gently cleanse the treated area with lukewarm water.

   Soak a cotton pad in lukewarm water and gently dab your eyebrows, avoiding any rubbing motions.

   Dry the area using a dry cotton pad, again with gentle dabbing to avoid friction.

   Repeat this process 4 times a day at regular intervals.

   For the first two weeks, avoid excessive moisture on the eyebrows (e.g., during baths or showers). After 7-14 days, when the initial healing has occurred, you may begin using a gentle micellar water for cleansing. Avoid products containing alcohol or harsh ingredients.

2. **Preventing Irritation**

   Do not scratch or rub your eyebrows, even if small scabs form. Allow the scabs to fall off naturally to avoid scarring or pigment loss.

   Avoid applying makeup to the eyebrow area until fully healed (approximately 7-14 days).

   For at least 14 days, avoid saunas, swimming pools, hot baths, and excessive sweating, as these can cause the pigment to fade or irritate the skin.

3. **Sun Protection**

   Avoid sun exposure and tanning beds for at least 4 weeks. UV radiation can cause the pigment to fade.

   Once your eyebrows are fully healed, apply a high SPF sunscreen to protect the pigment from fading.

4. **Avoiding Intensive Cosmetic Treatments**

   For 4-6 weeks post-procedure, avoid facial treatments such as chemical peels, laser treatments, or the use of strong creams around the eyebrow area, as these may weaken the pigment.

5. **Consulting a Specialist**

   If you have any concerns or notice unusual symptoms such as excessive redness, swelling, or oozing, contact the cosmetologist who performed the procedure.

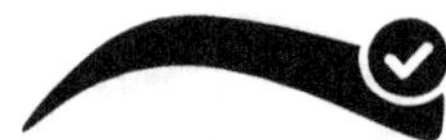

Healing process after micropigmentation

The healing process following permanent eyebrow makeup takes place in several stages and usually lasts between 4 to 6 weeks. During this time, the appearance of your eyebrows will change as the pigment gradually settles into the skin. Below are the stages of the healing process:

1. **Day 1: Immediately After the Procedure**
   Your eyebrows will look very intense, dark, and prominent. The skin may be slightly swollen and red. The pigment will appear darker than the final result, as the dye is still on the surface of the skin.

2. **Days 2–3**
   Swelling starts to subside, and the skin around the eyebrows may feel dry or tight.
   The eyebrows will still appear dark, but the skin begins to form a light protective layer.

3. **Days 4–7**
   Exfoliation begins. Scabs may form and fall off naturally, so it's important not to touch, scratch, or try to speed up the process.
   Your eyebrows may look uneven or have „empty" spots, but this is a normal part of healing as the pigment settles.

4. **Days 7–14**
   The scabs gradually fall off, and the pigment may look much lighter. Many people feel that their eyebrows are too light at this stage, but the color will continue to stabilize.
   Continue to avoid excessive washing and using cosmetics on the eyebrow area.

5. **Days 14–21**
   The eyebrows will appear lighter and more natural. Some areas may seem lighter than others, but this is part of the process.
   The pigment begins to settle into the skin, and the final color will start to become more visible.

6. **After 4 Weeks**
   By this point, the eyebrows are fully healed. The color will be 20-50% lighter compared to the first few days post-procedure.
   A touch-up session may be needed to fill any pigment gaps or refine the shape.

Date of your touch-up:

Post-procedure care after micropigmentation

Following a micropigmentation procedure, the skin requires special attention to ensure proper healing and long-lasting, aesthetic results. Below are the recommended post-care instructions:

1. **Hygiene**

   Always wash your hands before touching your eyebrows.

   For the first week, gently cleanse the treated area with lukewarm water.

   Soak a cotton pad in lukewarm water and gently dab your eyebrows, avoiding any rubbing motions.

   Dry the area using a dry cotton pad, again with gentle dabbing to avoid friction.

   Repeat this process 4 times a day at regular intervals.

   For the first two weeks, avoid excessive moisture on the eyebrows (e.g., during baths or showers). After 7-14 days, when the initial healing has occurred, you may begin using a gentle micellar water for cleansing. Avoid products containing alcohol or harsh ingredients.

2. **Preventing Irritation**

   Do not scratch or rub your eyebrows, even if small scabs form. Allow the scabs to fall off naturally to avoid scarring or pigment loss.

   Avoid applying makeup to the eyebrow area until fully healed (approximately 7-14 days).

   For at least 14 days, avoid saunas, swimming pools, hot baths, and excessive sweating, as these can cause the pigment to fade or irritate the skin.

3. **Sun Protection**

   Avoid sun exposure and tanning beds for at least 4 weeks. UV radiation can cause the pigment to fade.

   Once your eyebrows are fully healed, apply a high SPF sunscreen to protect the pigment from fading.

4. **Avoiding Intensive Cosmetic Treatments**

   For 4-6 weeks post-procedure, avoid facial treatments such as chemical peels, laser treatments, or the use of strong creams around the eyebrow area, as these may weaken the pigment.

5. **Consulting a Specialist**

   If you have any concerns or notice unusual symptoms such as excessive redness, swelling, or oozing, contact the cosmetologist who performed the procedure.

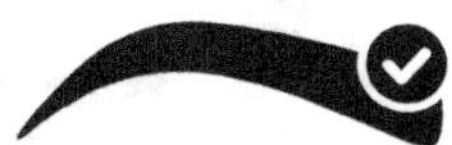

Healing process after micropigmentation

The healing process following permanent eyebrow makeup takes place in several stages and usually lasts between 4 to 6 weeks. During this time, the appearance of your eyebrows will change as the pigment gradually settles into the skin. Below are the stages of the healing process:

1. **Day 1: Immediately After the Procedure**
   Your eyebrows will look very intense, dark, and prominent. The skin may be slightly swollen and red. The pigment will appear darker than the final result, as the dye is still on the surface of the skin.

2. **Days 2–3**
   Swelling starts to subside, and the skin around the eyebrows may feel dry or tight.
   The eyebrows will still appear dark, but the skin begins to form a light protective layer.

3. **Days 4–7**
   Exfoliation begins. Scabs may form and fall off naturally, so it's important not to touch, scratch, or try to speed up the process.
   Your eyebrows may look uneven or have „empty" spots, but this is a normal part of healing as the pigment settles.

4. **Days 7–14**
   The scabs gradually fall off, and the pigment may look much lighter. Many people feel that their eyebrows are too light at this stage, but the color will continue to stabilize.
   Continue to avoid excessive washing and using cosmetics on the eyebrow area.

5. **Days 14–21**
   The eyebrows will appear lighter and more natural. Some areas may seem lighter than others, but this is part of the process.
   The pigment begins to settle into the skin, and the final color will start to become more visible.

6. **After 4 Weeks**
   By this point, the eyebrows are fully healed. The color will be 20-50% lighter compared to the first few days post-procedure.
   A touch-up session may be needed to fill any pigment gaps or refine the shape.

Date of your touch-up:

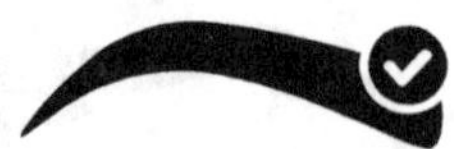

Post-procedure care after micropigmentation

Following a micropigmentation procedure, the skin requires special attention to ensure proper healing and long-lasting, aesthetic results. Below are the recommended post-care instructions:

1. **Hygiene**
   Always wash your hands before touching your eyebrows.
   For the first week, gently cleanse the treated area with lukewarm water.
   Soak a cotton pad in lukewarm water and gently dab your eyebrows, avoiding any rubbing motions.
   Dry the area using a dry cotton pad, again with gentle dabbing to avoid friction.
   Repeat this process 4 times a day at regular intervals.
   For the first two weeks, avoid excessive moisture on the eyebrows (e.g., during baths or showers). After 7-14 days, when the initial healing has occurred, you may begin using a gentle micellar water for cleansing. Avoid products containing alcohol or harsh ingredients.

2. **Preventing Irritation**
   Do not scratch or rub your eyebrows, even if small scabs form. Allow the scabs to fall off naturally to avoid scarring or pigment loss.
   Avoid applying makeup to the eyebrow area until fully healed (approximately 7-14 days).
   For at least 14 days, avoid saunas, swimming pools, hot baths, and excessive sweating, as these can cause the pigment to fade or irritate the skin.

3. **Sun Protection**
   Avoid sun exposure and tanning beds for at least 4 weeks. UV radiation can cause the pigment to fade.
   Once your eyebrows are fully healed, apply a high SPF sunscreen to protect the pigment from fading.

4. **Avoiding Intensive Cosmetic Treatments**
   For 4-6 weeks post-procedure, avoid facial treatments such as chemical peels, laser treatments, or the use of strong creams around the eyebrow area, as these may weaken the pigment.

5. **Consulting a Specialist**
   If you have any concerns or notice unusual symptoms such as excessive redness, swelling, or oozing, contact the cosmetologist who performed the procedure.

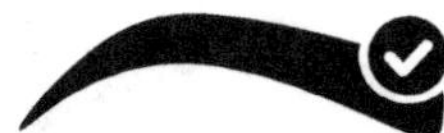

Healing process after micropigmentation

The healing process following permanent eyebrow makeup takes place in several stages and usually lasts between 4 to 6 weeks. During this time, the appearance of your eyebrows will change as the pigment gradually settles into the skin. Below are the stages of the healing process:

1. **Day 1: Immediately After the Procedure**
   Your eyebrows will look very intense, dark, and prominent. The skin may be slightly swollen and red. The pigment will appear darker than the final result, as the dye is still on the surface of the skin.

2. **Days 2–3**
   Swelling starts to subside, and the skin around the eyebrows may feel dry or tight.
   The eyebrows will still appear dark, but the skin begins to form a light protective layer.

3. **Days 4–7**
   Exfoliation begins. Scabs may form and fall off naturally, so it's important not to touch, scratch, or try to speed up the process.
   Your eyebrows may look uneven or have „empty" spots, but this is a normal part of healing as the pigment settles.

4. **Days 7–14**
   The scabs gradually fall off, and the pigment may look much lighter. Many people feel that their eyebrows are too light at this stage, but the color will continue to stabilize.
   Continue to avoid excessive washing and using cosmetics on the eyebrow area.

5. **Days 14–21**
   The eyebrows will appear lighter and more natural. Some areas may seem lighter than others, but this is part of the process.
   The pigment begins to settle into the skin, and the final color will start to become more visible.

6. **After 4 Weeks**
   By this point, the eyebrows are fully healed. The color will be 20-50% lighter compared to the first few days post-procedure.
   A touch-up session may be needed to fill any pigment gaps or refine the shape.

Date of your touch-up:

Post-procedure care after micropigmentation

Following a micropigmentation procedure, the skin requires special attention to ensure proper healing and long-lasting, aesthetic results. Below are the recommended post-care instructions:

1. **Hygiene**
   Always wash your hands before touching your eyebrows.
   For the first week, gently cleanse the treated area with lukewarm water.
   Soak a cotton pad in lukewarm water and gently dab your eyebrows, avoiding any rubbing motions.
   Dry the area using a dry cotton pad, again with gentle dabbing to avoid friction.
   Repeat this process 4 times a day at regular intervals.
   For the first two weeks, avoid excessive moisture on the eyebrows (e.g., during baths or showers). After 7-14 days, when the initial healing has occurred, you may begin using a gentle micellar water for cleansing. Avoid products containing alcohol or harsh ingredients.

2. **Preventing Irritation**
   Do not scratch or rub your eyebrows, even if small scabs form. Allow the scabs to fall off naturally to avoid scarring or pigment loss.
   Avoid applying makeup to the eyebrow area until fully healed (approximately 7-14 days).
   For at least 14 days, avoid saunas, swimming pools, hot baths, and excessive sweating, as these can cause the pigment to fade or irritate the skin.

3. **Sun Protection**
   Avoid sun exposure and tanning beds for at least 4 weeks. UV radiation can cause the pigment to fade.
   Once your eyebrows are fully healed, apply a high SPF sunscreen to protect the pigment from fading.

4. **Avoiding Intensive Cosmetic Treatments**
   For 4-6 weeks post-procedure, avoid facial treatments such as chemical peels, laser treatments, or the use of strong creams around the eyebrow area, as these may weaken the pigment.

5. **Consulting a Specialist**
   If you have any concerns or notice unusual symptoms such as excessive redness, swelling, or oozing, contact the cosmetologist who performed the procedure.

Healing process after micropigmentation

The healing process following permanent eyebrow makeup takes place in several stages and usually lasts between 4 to 6 weeks. During this time, the appearance of your eyebrows will change as the pigment gradually settles into the skin. Below are the stages of the healing process:

1. **Day 1: Immediately After the Procedure**
   Your eyebrows will look very intense, dark, and prominent. The skin may be slightly swollen and red. The pigment will appear darker than the final result, as the dye is still on the surface of the skin.

2. **Days 2–3**
   Swelling starts to subside, and the skin around the eyebrows may feel dry or tight.
   The eyebrows will still appear dark, but the skin begins to form a light protective layer.

3. **Days 4–7**
   Exfoliation begins. Scabs may form and fall off naturally, so it's important not to touch, scratch, or try to speed up the process.
   Your eyebrows may look uneven or have „empty" spots, but this is a normal part of healing as the pigment settles.

4. **Days 7–14**
   The scabs gradually fall off, and the pigment may look much lighter. Many people feel that their eyebrows are too light at this stage, but the color will continue to stabilize.
   Continue to avoid excessive washing and using cosmetics on the eyebrow area.

5. **Days 14–21**
   The eyebrows will appear lighter and more natural. Some areas may seem lighter than others, but this is part of the process.
   The pigment begins to settle into the skin, and the final color will start to become more visible.

6. **After 4 Weeks**
   By this point, the eyebrows are fully healed. The color will be 20-50% lighter compared to the first few days post-procedure.
   A touch-up session may be needed to fill any pigment gaps or refine the shape.

Date of your touch-up:

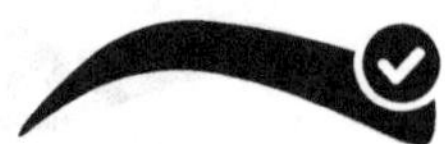

Post-procedure care after micropigmentation

Following a micropigmentation procedure, the skin requires special attention to ensure proper healing and long-lasting, aesthetic results. Below are the recommended post-care instructions:

1. **Hygiene**

   Always wash your hands before touching your eyebrows.

   For the first week, gently cleanse the treated area with lukewarm water.

   Soak a cotton pad in lukewarm water and gently dab your eyebrows, avoiding any rubbing motions.

   Dry the area using a dry cotton pad, again with gentle dabbing to avoid friction.

   Repeat this process 4 times a day at regular intervals.

   For the first two weeks, avoid excessive moisture on the eyebrows (e.g., during baths or showers). After 7-14 days, when the initial healing has occurred, you may begin using a gentle micellar water for cleansing. Avoid products containing alcohol or harsh ingredients.

2. **Preventing Irritation**

   Do not scratch or rub your eyebrows, even if small scabs form. Allow the scabs to fall off naturally to avoid scarring or pigment loss.

   Avoid applying makeup to the eyebrow area until fully healed (approximately 7-14 days).

   For at least 14 days, avoid saunas, swimming pools, hot baths, and excessive sweating, as these can cause the pigment to fade or irritate the skin.

3. **Sun Protection**

   Avoid sun exposure and tanning beds for at least 4 weeks. UV radiation can cause the pigment to fade.

   Once your eyebrows are fully healed, apply a high SPF sunscreen to protect the pigment from fading.

4. **Avoiding Intensive Cosmetic Treatments**

   For 4-6 weeks post-procedure, avoid facial treatments such as chemical peels, laser treatments, or the use of strong creams around the eyebrow area, as these may weaken the pigment.

5. **Consulting a Specialist**

   If you have any concerns or notice unusual symptoms such as excessive redness, swelling, or oozing, contact the cosmetologist who performed the procedure.

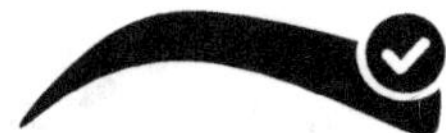

Healing process after micropigmentation

The healing process following permanent eyebrow makeup takes place in several stages and usually lasts between 4 to 6 weeks. During this time, the appearance of your eyebrows will change as the pigment gradually settles into the skin. Below are the stages of the healing process:

1. **Day 1: Immediately After the Procedure**
   Your eyebrows will look very intense, dark, and prominent. The skin may be slightly swollen and red. The pigment will appear darker than the final result, as the dye is still on the surface of the skin.

2. **Days 2–3**
   Swelling starts to subside, and the skin around the eyebrows may feel dry or tight.
   The eyebrows will still appear dark, but the skin begins to form a light protective layer.

3. **Days 4–7**
   Exfoliation begins. Scabs may form and fall off naturally, so it's important not to touch, scratch, or try to speed up the process.
   Your eyebrows may look uneven or have „empty" spots, but this is a normal part of healing as the pigment settles.

4. **Days 7–14**
   The scabs gradually fall off, and the pigment may look much lighter. Many people feel that their eyebrows are too light at this stage, but the color will continue to stabilize.
   Continue to avoid excessive washing and using cosmetics on the eyebrow area.

5. **Days 14–21**
   The eyebrows will appear lighter and more natural. Some areas may seem lighter than others, but this is part of the process.
   The pigment begins to settle into the skin, and the final color will start to become more visible.

6. **After 4 Weeks**
   By this point, the eyebrows are fully healed. The color will be 20-50% lighter compared to the first few days post-procedure.
   A touch-up session may be needed to fill any pigment gaps or refine the shape.

Date of your touch-up:

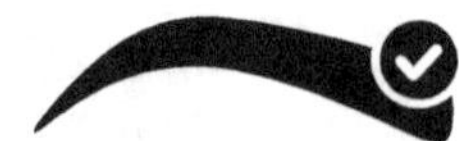

Post-procedure care after micropigmentation

Following a micropigmentation procedure, the skin requires special attention to ensure proper healing and long-lasting, aesthetic results. Below are the recommended post-care instructions:

1. **Hygiene**
   Always wash your hands before touching your eyebrows.
   For the first week, gently cleanse the treated area with lukewarm water.
   Soak a cotton pad in lukewarm water and gently dab your eyebrows, avoiding any rubbing motions.
   Dry the area using a dry cotton pad, again with gentle dabbing to avoid friction.
   Repeat this process 4 times a day at regular intervals.
   For the first two weeks, avoid excessive moisture on the eyebrows (e.g., during baths or showers). After 7-14 days, when the initial healing has occurred, you may begin using a gentle micellar water for cleansing. Avoid products containing alcohol or harsh ingredients.

2. **Preventing Irritation**
   Do not scratch or rub your eyebrows, even if small scabs form. Allow the scabs to fall off naturally to avoid scarring or pigment loss.
   Avoid applying makeup to the eyebrow area until fully healed (approximately 7-14 days).
   For at least 14 days, avoid saunas, swimming pools, hot baths, and excessive sweating, as these can cause the pigment to fade or irritate the skin.

3. **Sun Protection**
   Avoid sun exposure and tanning beds for at least 4 weeks. UV radiation can cause the pigment to fade.
   Once your eyebrows are fully healed, apply a high SPF sunscreen to protect the pigment from fading.

4. **Avoiding Intensive Cosmetic Treatments**
   For 4-6 weeks post-procedure, avoid facial treatments such as chemical peels, laser treatments, or the use of strong creams around the eyebrow area, as these may weaken the pigment.

5. **Consulting a Specialist**
   If you have any concerns or notice unusual symptoms such as excessive redness, swelling, or oozing, contact the cosmetologist who performed the procedure.

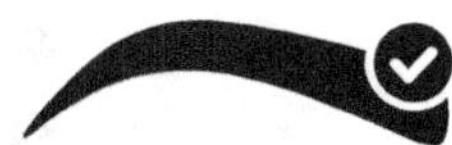

Healing process after micropigmentation

The healing process following permanent eyebrow makeup takes place in several stages and usually lasts between 4 to 6 weeks. During this time, the appearance of your eyebrows will change as the pigment gradually settles into the skin. Below are the stages of the healing process:

1. **Day 1: Immediately After the Procedure**
   Your eyebrows will look very intense, dark, and prominent. The skin may be slightly swollen and red. The pigment will appear darker than the final result, as the dye is still on the surface of the skin.

2. **Days 2–3**
   Swelling starts to subside, and the skin around the eyebrows may feel dry or tight.
   The eyebrows will still appear dark, but the skin begins to form a light protective layer.

3. **Days 4–7**
   Exfoliation begins. Scabs may form and fall off naturally, so it's important not to touch, scratch, or try to speed up the process.
   Your eyebrows may look uneven or have „empty" spots, but this is a normal part of healing as the pigment settles.

4. **Days 7–14**
   The scabs gradually fall off, and the pigment may look much lighter. Many people feel that their eyebrows are too light at this stage, but the color will continue to stabilize.
   Continue to avoid excessive washing and using cosmetics on the eyebrow area.

5. **Days 14–21**
   The eyebrows will appear lighter and more natural. Some areas may seem lighter than others, but this is part of the process.
   The pigment begins to settle into the skin, and the final color will start to become more visible.

6. **After 4 Weeks**
   By this point, the eyebrows are fully healed. The color will be 20-50% lighter compared to the first few days post-procedure.
   A touch-up session may be needed to fill any pigment gaps or refine the shape.

Date of your touch-up:

Post-procedure care after micropigmentation

Following a micropigmentation procedure, the skin requires special attention to ensure proper healing and long-lasting, aesthetic results. Below are the recommended post-care instructions:

1. **Hygiene**

   Always wash your hands before touching your eyebrows.

   For the first week, gently cleanse the treated area with lukewarm water.

   Soak a cotton pad in lukewarm water and gently dab your eyebrows, avoiding any rubbing motions.

   Dry the area using a dry cotton pad, again with gentle dabbing to avoid friction.

   Repeat this process 4 times a day at regular intervals.

   For the first two weeks, avoid excessive moisture on the eyebrows (e.g., during baths or showers). After 7-14 days, when the initial healing has occurred, you may begin using a gentle micellar water for cleansing. Avoid products containing alcohol or harsh ingredients.

2. **Preventing Irritation**

   Do not scratch or rub your eyebrows, even if small scabs form. Allow the scabs to fall off naturally to avoid scarring or pigment loss.

   Avoid applying makeup to the eyebrow area until fully healed (approximately 7-14 days).

   For at least 14 days, avoid saunas, swimming pools, hot baths, and excessive sweating, as these can cause the pigment to fade or irritate the skin.

3. **Sun Protection**

   Avoid sun exposure and tanning beds for at least 4 weeks. UV radiation can cause the pigment to fade.

   Once your eyebrows are fully healed, apply a high SPF sunscreen to protect the pigment from fading.

4. **Avoiding Intensive Cosmetic Treatments**

   For 4-6 weeks post-procedure, avoid facial treatments such as chemical peels, laser treatments, or the use of strong creams around the eyebrow area, as these may weaken the pigment.

5. **Consulting a Specialist**

   If you have any concerns or notice unusual symptoms such as excessive redness, swelling, or oozing, contact the cosmetologist who performed the procedure.

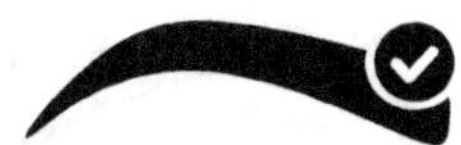

Healing process after micropigmentation

The healing process following permanent eyebrow makeup takes place in several stages and usually lasts between 4 to 6 weeks. During this time, the appearance of your eyebrows will change as the pigment gradually settles into the skin. Below are the stages of the healing process:

1. **Day 1: Immediately After the Procedure**
   Your eyebrows will look very intense, dark, and prominent. The skin may be slightly swollen and red. The pigment will appear darker than the final result, as the dye is still on the surface of the skin.

2. **Days 2–3**
   Swelling starts to subside, and the skin around the eyebrows may feel dry or tight.
   The eyebrows will still appear dark, but the skin begins to form a light protective layer.

3. **Days 4–7**
   Exfoliation begins. Scabs may form and fall off naturally, so it's important not to touch, scratch, or try to speed up the process.
   Your eyebrows may look uneven or have „empty" spots, but this is a normal part of healing as the pigment settles.

4. **Days 7–14**
   The scabs gradually fall off, and the pigment may look much lighter. Many people feel that their eyebrows are too light at this stage, but the color will continue to stabilize.
   Continue to avoid excessive washing and using cosmetics on the eyebrow area.

5. **Days 14–21**
   The eyebrows will appear lighter and more natural. Some areas may seem lighter than others, but this is part of the process.
   The pigment begins to settle into the skin, and the final color will start to become more visible.

6. **After 4 Weeks**
   By this point, the eyebrows are fully healed. The color will be 20-50% lighter compared to the first few days post-procedure.
   A touch-up session may be needed to fill any pigment gaps or refine the shape.

Date of your touch-up:

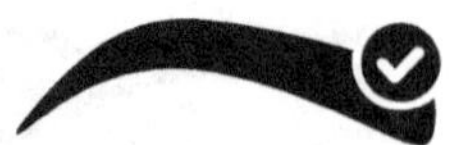

Post-procedure care after micropigmentation

Following a micropigmentation procedure, the skin requires special attention to ensure proper healing and long-lasting, aesthetic results. Below are the recommended post-care instructions:

1. **Hygiene**

   Always wash your hands before touching your eyebrows.

   For the first week, gently cleanse the treated area with lukewarm water.

   Soak a cotton pad in lukewarm water and gently dab your eyebrows, avoiding any rubbing motions.

   Dry the area using a dry cotton pad, again with gentle dabbing to avoid friction.

   Repeat this process 4 times a day at regular intervals.

   For the first two weeks, avoid excessive moisture on the eyebrows (e.g., during baths or showers). After 7-14 days, when the initial healing has occurred, you may begin using a gentle micellar water for cleansing. Avoid products containing alcohol or harsh ingredients.

2. **Preventing Irritation**

   Do not scratch or rub your eyebrows, even if small scabs form. Allow the scabs to fall off naturally to avoid scarring or pigment loss.

   Avoid applying makeup to the eyebrow area until fully healed (approximately 7-14 days).

   For at least 14 days, avoid saunas, swimming pools, hot baths, and excessive sweating, as these can cause the pigment to fade or irritate the skin.

3. **Sun Protection**

   Avoid sun exposure and tanning beds for at least 4 weeks. UV radiation can cause the pigment to fade.

   Once your eyebrows are fully healed, apply a high SPF sunscreen to protect the pigment from fading.

4. **Avoiding Intensive Cosmetic Treatments**

   For 4-6 weeks post-procedure, avoid facial treatments such as chemical peels, laser treatments, or the use of strong creams around the eyebrow area, as these may weaken the pigment.

5. **Consulting a Specialist**

   If you have any concerns or notice unusual symptoms such as excessive redness, swelling, or oozing, contact the cosmetologist who performed the procedure.

Healing process after micropigmentation

The healing process following permanent eyebrow makeup takes place in several stages and usually lasts between 4 to 6 weeks. During this time, the appearance of your eyebrows will change as the pigment gradually settles into the skin. Below are the stages of the healing process:

1. **Day 1: Immediately After the Procedure**
   Your eyebrows will look very intense, dark, and prominent. The skin may be slightly swollen and red. The pigment will appear darker than the final result, as the dye is still on the surface of the skin.

2. **Days 2–3**
   Swelling starts to subside, and the skin around the eyebrows may feel dry or tight.
   The eyebrows will still appear dark, but the skin begins to form a light protective layer.

3. **Days 4–7**
   Exfoliation begins. Scabs may form and fall off naturally, so it's important not to touch, scratch, or try to speed up the process.
   Your eyebrows may look uneven or have „empty" spots, but this is a normal part of healing as the pigment settles.

4. **Days 7–14**
   The scabs gradually fall off, and the pigment may look much lighter. Many people feel that their eyebrows are too light at this stage, but the color will continue to stabilize.
   Continue to avoid excessive washing and using cosmetics on the eyebrow area.

5. **Days 14–21**
   The eyebrows will appear lighter and more natural. Some areas may seem lighter than others, but this is part of the process.
   The pigment begins to settle into the skin, and the final color will start to become more visible.

6. **After 4 Weeks**
   By this point, the eyebrows are fully healed. The color will be 20-50% lighter compared to the first few days post-procedure.
   A touch-up session may be needed to fill any pigment gaps or refine the shape.

Date of your touch-up:

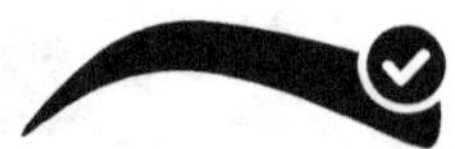

Post-procedure care after micropigmentation

Following a micropigmentation procedure, the skin requires special attention to ensure proper healing and long-lasting, aesthetic results. Below are the recommended post-care instructions:

1. **Hygiene**

   Always wash your hands before touching your eyebrows.

   For the first week, gently cleanse the treated area with lukewarm water.

   Soak a cotton pad in lukewarm water and gently dab your eyebrows, avoiding any rubbing motions.

   Dry the area using a dry cotton pad, again with gentle dabbing to avoid friction.

   Repeat this process 4 times a day at regular intervals.

   For the first two weeks, avoid excessive moisture on the eyebrows (e.g., during baths or showers). After 7-14 days, when the initial healing has occurred, you may begin using a gentle micellar water for cleansing. Avoid products containing alcohol or harsh ingredients.

2. **Preventing Irritation**

   Do not scratch or rub your eyebrows, even if small scabs form. Allow the scabs to fall off naturally to avoid scarring or pigment loss.

   Avoid applying makeup to the eyebrow area until fully healed (approximately 7-14 days).

   For at least 14 days, avoid saunas, swimming pools, hot baths, and excessive sweating, as these can cause the pigment to fade or irritate the skin.

3. **Sun Protection**

   Avoid sun exposure and tanning beds for at least 4 weeks. UV radiation can cause the pigment to fade.

   Once your eyebrows are fully healed, apply a high SPF sunscreen to protect the pigment from fading.

4. **Avoiding Intensive Cosmetic Treatments**

   For 4-6 weeks post-procedure, avoid facial treatments such as chemical peels, laser treatments, or the use of strong creams around the eyebrow area, as these may weaken the pigment.

5. **Consulting a Specialist**

   If you have any concerns or notice unusual symptoms such as excessive redness, swelling, or oozing, contact the cosmetologist who performed the procedure.

Healing process after micropigmentation

The healing process following permanent eyebrow makeup takes place in several stages and usually lasts between 4 to 6 weeks. During this time, the appearance of your eyebrows will change as the pigment gradually settles into the skin. Below are the stages of the healing process:

1. **Day 1: Immediately After the Procedure**
   Your eyebrows will look very intense, dark, and prominent. The skin may be slightly swollen and red. The pigment will appear darker than the final result, as the dye is still on the surface of the skin.

2. **Days 2–3**
   Swelling starts to subside, and the skin around the eyebrows may feel dry or tight.
   The eyebrows will still appear dark, but the skin begins to form a light protective layer.

3. **Days 4–7**
   Exfoliation begins. Scabs may form and fall off naturally, so it's important not to touch, scratch, or try to speed up the process.
   Your eyebrows may look uneven or have „empty" spots, but this is a normal part of healing as the pigment settles.

4. **Days 7–14**
   The scabs gradually fall off, and the pigment may look much lighter. Many people feel that their eyebrows are too light at this stage, but the color will continue to stabilize.
   Continue to avoid excessive washing and using cosmetics on the eyebrow area.

5. **Days 14–21**
   The eyebrows will appear lighter and more natural. Some areas may seem lighter than others, but this is part of the process.
   The pigment begins to settle into the skin, and the final color will start to become more visible.

6. **After 4 Weeks**
   By this point, the eyebrows are fully healed. The color will be 20-50% lighter compared to the first few days post-procedure.
   A touch-up session may be needed to fill any pigment gaps or refine the shape.

Date of your touch-up:

Post-procedure care after micropigmentation

Following a micropigmentation procedure, the skin requires special attention to ensure proper healing and long-lasting, aesthetic results. Below are the recommended post-care instructions:

1. **Hygiene**

   Always wash your hands before touching your eyebrows.

   For the first week, gently cleanse the treated area with lukewarm water.

   Soak a cotton pad in lukewarm water and gently dab your eyebrows, avoiding any rubbing motions.

   Dry the area using a dry cotton pad, again with gentle dabbing to avoid friction.

   Repeat this process 4 times a day at regular intervals.

   For the first two weeks, avoid excessive moisture on the eyebrows (e.g., during baths or showers). After 7-14 days, when the initial healing has occurred, you may begin using a gentle micellar water for cleansing. Avoid products containing alcohol or harsh ingredients.

2. **Preventing Irritation**

   Do not scratch or rub your eyebrows, even if small scabs form. Allow the scabs to fall off naturally to avoid scarring or pigment loss.

   Avoid applying makeup to the eyebrow area until fully healed (approximately 7-14 days).

   For at least 14 days, avoid saunas, swimming pools, hot baths, and excessive sweating, as these can cause the pigment to fade or irritate the skin.

3. **Sun Protection**

   Avoid sun exposure and tanning beds for at least 4 weeks. UV radiation can cause the pigment to fade.

   Once your eyebrows are fully healed, apply a high SPF sunscreen to protect the pigment from fading.

4. **Avoiding Intensive Cosmetic Treatments**

   For 4-6 weeks post-procedure, avoid facial treatments such as chemical peels, laser treatments, or the use of strong creams around the eyebrow area, as these may weaken the pigment.

5. **Consulting a Specialist**

   If you have any concerns or notice unusual symptoms such as excessive redness, swelling, or oozing, contact the cosmetologist who performed the procedure.

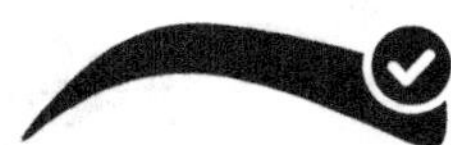

Healing process after micropigmentation

The healing process following permanent eyebrow makeup takes place in several stages and usually lasts between 4 to 6 weeks. During this time, the appearance of your eyebrows will change as the pigment gradually settles into the skin. Below are the stages of the healing process:

1. **Day 1: Immediately After the Procedure**
   Your eyebrows will look very intense, dark, and prominent. The skin may be slightly swollen and red. The pigment will appear darker than the final result, as the dye is still on the surface of the skin.

2. **Days 2–3**
   Swelling starts to subside, and the skin around the eyebrows may feel dry or tight.
   The eyebrows will still appear dark, but the skin begins to form a light protective layer.

3. **Days 4–7**
   Exfoliation begins. Scabs may form and fall off naturally, so it's important not to touch, scratch, or try to speed up the process.
   Your eyebrows may look uneven or have „empty" spots, but this is a normal part of healing as the pigment settles.

4. **Days 7–14**
   The scabs gradually fall off, and the pigment may look much lighter. Many people feel that their eyebrows are too light at this stage, but the color will continue to stabilize.
   Continue to avoid excessive washing and using cosmetics on the eyebrow area.

5. **Days 14–21**
   The eyebrows will appear lighter and more natural. Some areas may seem lighter than others, but this is part of the process.
   The pigment begins to settle into the skin, and the final color will start to become more visible.

6. **After 4 Weeks**
   By this point, the eyebrows are fully healed. The color will be 20-50% lighter compared to the first few days post-procedure.
   A touch-up session may be needed to fill any pigment gaps or refine the shape.

Date of your touch-up:

Post-procedure care after micropigmentation

Following a micropigmentation procedure, the skin requires special attention to ensure proper healing and long-lasting, aesthetic results. Below are the recommended post-care instructions:

1. **Hygiene**

   Always wash your hands before touching your eyebrows.

   For the first week, gently cleanse the treated area with lukewarm water.

   Soak a cotton pad in lukewarm water and gently dab your eyebrows, avoiding any rubbing motions.

   Dry the area using a dry cotton pad, again with gentle dabbing to avoid friction.

   Repeat this process 4 times a day at regular intervals.

   For the first two weeks, avoid excessive moisture on the eyebrows (e.g., during baths or showers). After 7-14 days, when the initial healing has occurred, you may begin using a gentle micellar water for cleansing. Avoid products containing alcohol or harsh ingredients.

2. **Preventing Irritation**

   Do not scratch or rub your eyebrows, even if small scabs form. Allow the scabs to fall off naturally to avoid scarring or pigment loss.

   Avoid applying makeup to the eyebrow area until fully healed (approximately 7-14 days).

   For at least 14 days, avoid saunas, swimming pools, hot baths, and excessive sweating, as these can cause the pigment to fade or irritate the skin.

3. **Sun Protection**

   Avoid sun exposure and tanning beds for at least 4 weeks. UV radiation can cause the pigment to fade.

   Once your eyebrows are fully healed, apply a high SPF sunscreen to protect the pigment from fading.

4. **Avoiding Intensive Cosmetic Treatments**

   For 4-6 weeks post-procedure, avoid facial treatments such as chemical peels, laser treatments, or the use of strong creams around the eyebrow area, as these may weaken the pigment.

5. **Consulting a Specialist**

   If you have any concerns or notice unusual symptoms such as excessive redness, swelling, or oozing, contact the cosmetologist who performed the procedure.

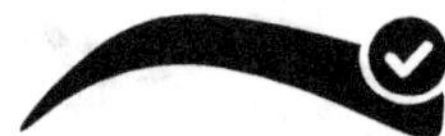

Healing process after micropigmentation

The healing process following permanent eyebrow makeup takes place in several stages and usually lasts between 4 to 6 weeks. During this time, the appearance of your eyebrows will change as the pigment gradually settles into the skin. Below are the stages of the healing process:

1. **Day 1: Immediately After the Procedure**
   Your eyebrows will look very intense, dark, and prominent. The skin may be slightly swollen and red. The pigment will appear darker than the final result, as the dye is still on the surface of the skin.

2. **Days 2–3**
   Swelling starts to subside, and the skin around the eyebrows may feel dry or tight.
   The eyebrows will still appear dark, but the skin begins to form a light protective layer.

3. **Days 4–7**
   Exfoliation begins. Scabs may form and fall off naturally, so it's important not to touch, scratch, or try to speed up the process.
   Your eyebrows may look uneven or have „empty" spots, but this is a normal part of healing as the pigment settles.

4. **Days 7–14**
   The scabs gradually fall off, and the pigment may look much lighter. Many people feel that their eyebrows are too light at this stage, but the color will continue to stabilize.
   Continue to avoid excessive washing and using cosmetics on the eyebrow area.

5. **Days 14–21**
   The eyebrows will appear lighter and more natural. Some areas may seem lighter than others, but this is part of the process.
   The pigment begins to settle into the skin, and the final color will start to become more visible.

6. **After 4 Weeks**
   By this point, the eyebrows are fully healed. The color will be 20-50% lighter compared to the first few days post-procedure.
   A touch-up session may be needed to fill any pigment gaps or refine the shape.

Date of your touch-up:

Post-procedure care after micropigmentation

Following a micropigmentation procedure, the skin requires special attention to ensure proper healing and long-lasting, aesthetic results. Below are the recommended post-care instructions:

1. **Hygiene**

   Always wash your hands before touching your eyebrows.

   For the first week, gently cleanse the treated area with lukewarm water.

   Soak a cotton pad in lukewarm water and gently dab your eyebrows, avoiding any rubbing motions.

   Dry the area using a dry cotton pad, again with gentle dabbing to avoid friction.

   Repeat this process 4 times a day at regular intervals.

   For the first two weeks, avoid excessive moisture on the eyebrows (e.g., during baths or showers). After 7-14 days, when the initial healing has occurred, you may begin using a gentle micellar water for cleansing. Avoid products containing alcohol or harsh ingredients.

2. **Preventing Irritation**

   Do not scratch or rub your eyebrows, even if small scabs form. Allow the scabs to fall off naturally to avoid scarring or pigment loss.

   Avoid applying makeup to the eyebrow area until fully healed (approximately 7-14 days).

   For at least 14 days, avoid saunas, swimming pools, hot baths, and excessive sweating, as these can cause the pigment to fade or irritate the skin.

3. **Sun Protection**

   Avoid sun exposure and tanning beds for at least 4 weeks. UV radiation can cause the pigment to fade.

   Once your eyebrows are fully healed, apply a high SPF sunscreen to protect the pigment from fading.

4. **Avoiding Intensive Cosmetic Treatments**

   For 4-6 weeks post-procedure, avoid facial treatments such as chemical peels, laser treatments, or the use of strong creams around the eyebrow area, as these may weaken the pigment.

5. **Consulting a Specialist**

   If you have any concerns or notice unusual symptoms such as excessive redness, swelling, or oozing, contact the cosmetologist who performed the procedure.

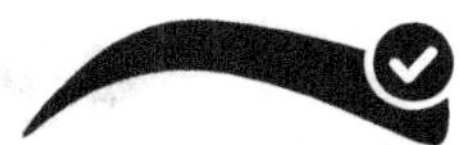

Healing process after micropigmentation

The healing process following permanent eyebrow makeup takes place in several stages and usually lasts between 4 to 6 weeks. During this time, the appearance of your eyebrows will change as the pigment gradually settles into the skin. Below are the stages of the healing process:

1. **Day 1: Immediately After the Procedure**
   Your eyebrows will look very intense, dark, and prominent. The skin may be slightly swollen and red. The pigment will appear darker than the final result, as the dye is still on the surface of the skin.

2. **Days 2–3**
   Swelling starts to subside, and the skin around the eyebrows may feel dry or tight.
   The eyebrows will still appear dark, but the skin begins to form a light protective layer.

3. **Days 4–7**
   Exfoliation begins. Scabs may form and fall off naturally, so it's important not to touch, scratch, or try to speed up the process.
   Your eyebrows may look uneven or have „empty" spots, but this is a normal part of healing as the pigment settles.

4. **Days 7–14**
   The scabs gradually fall off, and the pigment may look much lighter. Many people feel that their eyebrows are too light at this stage, but the color will continue to stabilize.
   Continue to avoid excessive washing and using cosmetics on the eyebrow area.

5. **Days 14–21**
   The eyebrows will appear lighter and more natural. Some areas may seem lighter than others, but this is part of the process.
   The pigment begins to settle into the skin, and the final color will start to become more visible.

6. **After 4 Weeks**
   By this point, the eyebrows are fully healed. The color will be 20-50% lighter compared to the first few days post-procedure.
   A touch-up session may be needed to fill any pigment gaps or refine the shape.

Date of your touch-up:

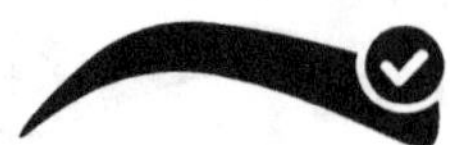

Post-procedure care after micropigmentation

Following a micropigmentation procedure, the skin requires special attention to ensure proper healing and long-lasting, aesthetic results. Below are the recommended post-care instructions:

1. **Hygiene**
   Always wash your hands before touching your eyebrows.
   For the first week, gently cleanse the treated area with lukewarm water.
   Soak a cotton pad in lukewarm water and gently dab your eyebrows, avoiding any rubbing motions.
   Dry the area using a dry cotton pad, again with gentle dabbing to avoid friction.
   Repeat this process 4 times a day at regular intervals.
   For the first two weeks, avoid excessive moisture on the eyebrows (e.g., during baths or showers). After 7-14 days, when the initial healing has occurred, you may begin using a gentle micellar water for cleansing. Avoid products containing alcohol or harsh ingredients.

2. **Preventing Irritation**
   Do not scratch or rub your eyebrows, even if small scabs form. Allow the scabs to fall off naturally to avoid scarring or pigment loss.
   Avoid applying makeup to the eyebrow area until fully healed (approximately 7-14 days).
   For at least 14 days, avoid saunas, swimming pools, hot baths, and excessive sweating, as these can cause the pigment to fade or irritate the skin.

3. **Sun Protection**
   Avoid sun exposure and tanning beds for at least 4 weeks. UV radiation can cause the pigment to fade.
   Once your eyebrows are fully healed, apply a high SPF sunscreen to protect the pigment from fading.

4. **Avoiding Intensive Cosmetic Treatments**
   For 4-6 weeks post-procedure, avoid facial treatments such as chemical peels, laser treatments, or the use of strong creams around the eyebrow area, as these may weaken the pigment.

5. **Consulting a Specialist**
   If you have any concerns or notice unusual symptoms such as excessive redness, swelling, or oozing, contact the cosmetologist who performed the procedure.

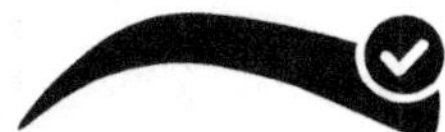

Healing process after micropigmentation

The healing process following permanent eyebrow makeup takes place in several stages and usually lasts between 4 to 6 weeks. During this time, the appearance of your eyebrows will change as the pigment gradually settles into the skin. Below are the stages of the healing process:

1. **Day 1: Immediately After the Procedure**
   Your eyebrows will look very intense, dark, and prominent. The skin may be slightly swollen and red. The pigment will appear darker than the final result, as the dye is still on the surface of the skin.

2. **Days 2–3**
   Swelling starts to subside, and the skin around the eyebrows may feel dry or tight.
   The eyebrows will still appear dark, but the skin begins to form a light protective layer.

3. **Days 4–7**
   Exfoliation begins. Scabs may form and fall off naturally, so it's important not to touch, scratch, or try to speed up the process.
   Your eyebrows may look uneven or have „empty" spots, but this is a normal part of healing as the pigment settles.

4. **Days 7–14**
   The scabs gradually fall off, and the pigment may look much lighter. Many people feel that their eyebrows are too light at this stage, but the color will continue to stabilize.
   Continue to avoid excessive washing and using cosmetics on the eyebrow area.

5. **Days 14–21**
   The eyebrows will appear lighter and more natural. Some areas may seem lighter than others, but this is part of the process.
   The pigment begins to settle into the skin, and the final color will start to become more visible.

6. **After 4 Weeks**
   By this point, the eyebrows are fully healed. The color will be 20-50% lighter compared to the first few days post-procedure.
   A touch-up session may be needed to fill any pigment gaps or refine the shape.

Date of your touch-up:

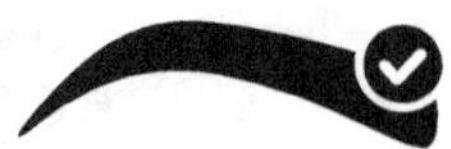

Post-procedure care after micropigmentation

Following a micropigmentation procedure, the skin requires special attention to ensure proper healing and long-lasting, aesthetic results. Below are the recommended post-care instructions:

1. **Hygiene**

   Always wash your hands before touching your eyebrows.

   For the first week, gently cleanse the treated area with lukewarm water.

   Soak a cotton pad in lukewarm water and gently dab your eyebrows, avoiding any rubbing motions.

   Dry the area using a dry cotton pad, again with gentle dabbing to avoid friction.

   Repeat this process 4 times a day at regular intervals.

   For the first two weeks, avoid excessive moisture on the eyebrows (e.g., during baths or showers). After 7-14 days, when the initial healing has occurred, you may begin using a gentle micellar water for cleansing. Avoid products containing alcohol or harsh ingredients.

2. **Preventing Irritation**

   Do not scratch or rub your eyebrows, even if small scabs form. Allow the scabs to fall off naturally to avoid scarring or pigment loss.

   Avoid applying makeup to the eyebrow area until fully healed (approximately 7-14 days).

   For at least 14 days, avoid saunas, swimming pools, hot baths, and excessive sweating, as these can cause the pigment to fade or irritate the skin.

3. **Sun Protection**

   Avoid sun exposure and tanning beds for at least 4 weeks. UV radiation can cause the pigment to fade.

   Once your eyebrows are fully healed, apply a high SPF sunscreen to protect the pigment from fading.

4. **Avoiding Intensive Cosmetic Treatments**

   For 4-6 weeks post-procedure, avoid facial treatments such as chemical peels, laser treatments, or the use of strong creams around the eyebrow area, as these may weaken the pigment.

5. **Consulting a Specialist**

   If you have any concerns or notice unusual symptoms such as excessive redness, swelling, or oozing, contact the cosmetologist who performed the procedure.

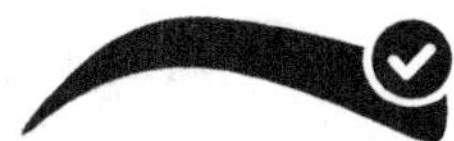

Healing process after micropigmentation

The healing process following permanent eyebrow makeup takes place in several stages and usually lasts between 4 to 6 weeks. During this time, the appearance of your eyebrows will change as the pigment gradually settles into the skin. Below are the stages of the healing process:

1. **Day 1: Immediately After the Procedure**
   Your eyebrows will look very intense, dark, and prominent. The skin may be slightly swollen and red. The pigment will appear darker than the final result, as the dye is still on the surface of the skin.

2. **Days 2–3**
   Swelling starts to subside, and the skin around the eyebrows may feel dry or tight.
   The eyebrows will still appear dark, but the skin begins to form a light protective layer.

3. **Days 4–7**
   Exfoliation begins. Scabs may form and fall off naturally, so it's important not to touch, scratch, or try to speed up the process.
   Your eyebrows may look uneven or have „empty" spots, but this is a normal part of healing as the pigment settles.

4. **Days 7–14**
   The scabs gradually fall off, and the pigment may look much lighter. Many people feel that their eyebrows are too light at this stage, but the color will continue to stabilize.
   Continue to avoid excessive washing and using cosmetics on the eyebrow area.

5. **Days 14–21**
   The eyebrows will appear lighter and more natural. Some areas may seem lighter than others, but this is part of the process.
   The pigment begins to settle into the skin, and the final color will start to become more visible.

6. **After 4 Weeks**
   By this point, the eyebrows are fully healed. The color will be 20-50% lighter compared to the first few days post-procedure.
   A touch-up session may be needed to fill any pigment gaps or refine the shape.

Date of your touch-up:

Post-procedure care after micropigmentation

Following a micropigmentation procedure, the skin requires special attention to ensure proper healing and long-lasting, aesthetic results. Below are the recommended post-care instructions:

1. **Hygiene**
   Always wash your hands before touching your eyebrows.
   For the first week, gently cleanse the treated area with lukewarm water.
   Soak a cotton pad in lukewarm water and gently dab your eyebrows, avoiding any rubbing motions.
   Dry the area using a dry cotton pad, again with gentle dabbing to avoid friction.
   Repeat this process 4 times a day at regular intervals.
   For the first two weeks, avoid excessive moisture on the eyebrows (e.g., during baths or showers). After 7-14 days, when the initial healing has occurred, you may begin using a gentle micellar water for cleansing. Avoid products containing alcohol or harsh ingredients.

2. **Preventing Irritation**
   Do not scratch or rub your eyebrows, even if small scabs form. Allow the scabs to fall off naturally to avoid scarring or pigment loss.
   Avoid applying makeup to the eyebrow area until fully healed (approximately 7-14 days).
   For at least 14 days, avoid saunas, swimming pools, hot baths, and excessive sweating, as these can cause the pigment to fade or irritate the skin.

3. **Sun Protection**
   Avoid sun exposure and tanning beds for at least 4 weeks. UV radiation can cause the pigment to fade.
   Once your eyebrows are fully healed, apply a high SPF sunscreen to protect the pigment from fading.

4. **Avoiding Intensive Cosmetic Treatments**
   For 4-6 weeks post-procedure, avoid facial treatments such as chemical peels, laser treatments, or the use of strong creams around the eyebrow area, as these may weaken the pigment.

5. **Consulting a Specialist**
   If you have any concerns or notice unusual symptoms such as excessive redness, swelling, or oozing, contact the cosmetologist who performed the procedure.

Healing process after micropigmentation

The healing process following permanent eyebrow makeup takes place in several stages and usually lasts between 4 to 6 weeks. During this time, the appearance of your eyebrows will change as the pigment gradually settles into the skin. Below are the stages of the healing process:

1. **Day 1: Immediately After the Procedure**

   Your eyebrows will look very intense, dark, and prominent. The skin may be slightly swollen and red. The pigment will appear darker than the final result, as the dye is still on the surface of the skin.

2. **Days 2–3**

   Swelling starts to subside, and the skin around the eyebrows may feel dry or tight.
   The eyebrows will still appear dark, but the skin begins to form a light protective layer.

3. **Days 4–7**

   Exfoliation begins. Scabs may form and fall off naturally, so it's important not to touch, scratch, or try to speed up the process.
   Your eyebrows may look uneven or have „empty" spots, but this is a normal part of healing as the pigment settles.

4. **Days 7–14**

   The scabs gradually fall off, and the pigment may look much lighter. Many people feel that their eyebrows are too light at this stage, but the color will continue to stabilize.
   Continue to avoid excessive washing and using cosmetics on the eyebrow area.

5. **Days 14–21**

   The eyebrows will appear lighter and more natural. Some areas may seem lighter than others, but this is part of the process.
   The pigment begins to settle into the skin, and the final color will start to become more visible.

6. **After 4 Weeks**

   By this point, the eyebrows are fully healed. The color will be 20-50% lighter compared to the first few days post-procedure.
   A touch-up session may be needed to fill any pigment gaps or refine the shape.

Date of your touch-up:

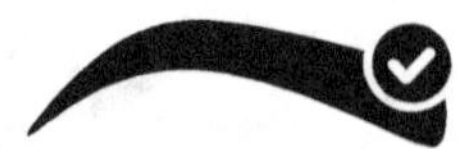

Post-procedure care after micropigmentation

Following a micropigmentation procedure, the skin requires special attention to ensure proper healing and long-lasting, aesthetic results. Below are the recommended post-care instructions:

1. **Hygiene**
   Always wash your hands before touching your eyebrows.
   For the first week, gently cleanse the treated area with lukewarm water.
   Soak a cotton pad in lukewarm water and gently dab your eyebrows, avoiding any rubbing motions.
   Dry the area using a dry cotton pad, again with gentle dabbing to avoid friction.
   Repeat this process 4 times a day at regular intervals.
   For the first two weeks, avoid excessive moisture on the eyebrows (e.g., during baths or showers). After 7-14 days, when the initial healing has occurred, you may begin using a gentle micellar water for cleansing. Avoid products containing alcohol or harsh ingredients.

2. **Preventing Irritation**
   Do not scratch or rub your eyebrows, even if small scabs form. Allow the scabs to fall off naturally to avoid scarring or pigment loss.
   Avoid applying makeup to the eyebrow area until fully healed (approximately 7-14 days).
   For at least 14 days, avoid saunas, swimming pools, hot baths, and excessive sweating, as these can cause the pigment to fade or irritate the skin.

3. **Sun Protection**
   Avoid sun exposure and tanning beds for at least 4 weeks. UV radiation can cause the pigment to fade.
   Once your eyebrows are fully healed, apply a high SPF sunscreen to protect the pigment from fading.

4. **Avoiding Intensive Cosmetic Treatments**
   For 4-6 weeks post-procedure, avoid facial treatments such as chemical peels, laser treatments, or the use of strong creams around the eyebrow area, as these may weaken the pigment.

5. **Consulting a Specialist**
   If you have any concerns or notice unusual symptoms such as excessive redness, swelling, or oozing, contact the cosmetologist who performed the procedure.

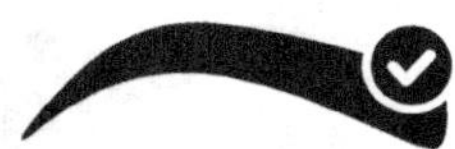

Healing process after micropigmentation

The healing process following permanent eyebrow makeup takes place in several stages and usually lasts between 4 to 6 weeks. During this time, the appearance of your eyebrows will change as the pigment gradually settles into the skin. Below are the stages of the healing process:

1. **Day 1: Immediately After the Procedure**
   Your eyebrows will look very intense, dark, and prominent. The skin may be slightly swollen and red. The pigment will appear darker than the final result, as the dye is still on the surface of the skin.

2. **Days 2–3**
   Swelling starts to subside, and the skin around the eyebrows may feel dry or tight.
   The eyebrows will still appear dark, but the skin begins to form a light protective layer.

3. **Days 4–7**
   Exfoliation begins. Scabs may form and fall off naturally, so it's important not to touch, scratch, or try to speed up the process.
   Your eyebrows may look uneven or have „empty" spots, but this is a normal part of healing as the pigment settles.

4. **Days 7–14**
   The scabs gradually fall off, and the pigment may look much lighter. Many people feel that their eyebrows are too light at this stage, but the color will continue to stabilize.
   Continue to avoid excessive washing and using cosmetics on the eyebrow area.

5. **Days 14–21**
   The eyebrows will appear lighter and more natural. Some areas may seem lighter than others, but this is part of the process.
   The pigment begins to settle into the skin, and the final color will start to become more visible.

6. **After 4 Weeks**
   By this point, the eyebrows are fully healed. The color will be 20-50% lighter compared to the first few days post-procedure.
   A touch-up session may be needed to fill any pigment gaps or refine the shape.

Date of your touch-up:

Post-procedure care after micropigmentation

Following a micropigmentation procedure, the skin requires special attention to ensure proper healing and long-lasting, aesthetic results. Below are the recommended post-care instructions:

1. **Hygiene**

   Always wash your hands before touching your eyebrows.
   For the first week, gently cleanse the treated area with lukewarm water.
   Soak a cotton pad in lukewarm water and gently dab your eyebrows, avoiding any rubbing motions.
   Dry the area using a dry cotton pad, again with gentle dabbing to avoid friction.
   Repeat this process 4 times a day at regular intervals.
   For the first two weeks, avoid excessive moisture on the eyebrows (e.g., during baths or showers). After 7-14 days, when the initial healing has occurred, you may begin using a gentle micellar water for cleansing. Avoid products containing alcohol or harsh ingredients.

2. **Preventing Irritation**

   Do not scratch or rub your eyebrows, even if small scabs form. Allow the scabs to fall off naturally to avoid scarring or pigment loss.
   Avoid applying makeup to the eyebrow area until fully healed (approximately 7-14 days).
   For at least 14 days, avoid saunas, swimming pools, hot baths, and excessive sweating, as these can cause the pigment to fade or irritate the skin.

3. **Sun Protection**

   Avoid sun exposure and tanning beds for at least 4 weeks. UV radiation can cause the pigment to fade.
   Once your eyebrows are fully healed, apply a high SPF sunscreen to protect the pigment from fading.

4. **Avoiding Intensive Cosmetic Treatments**

   For 4-6 weeks post-procedure, avoid facial treatments such as chemical peels, laser treatments, or the use of strong creams around the eyebrow area, as these may weaken the pigment.

5. **Consulting a Specialist**

   If you have any concerns or notice unusual symptoms such as excessive redness, swelling, or oozing, contact the cosmetologist who performed the procedure.

Healing process after micropigmentation

The healing process following permanent eyebrow makeup takes place in several stages and usually lasts between 4 to 6 weeks. During this time, the appearance of your eyebrows will change as the pigment gradually settles into the skin. Below are the stages of the healing process:

1. **Day 1: Immediately After the Procedure**
   Your eyebrows will look very intense, dark, and prominent. The skin may be slightly swollen and red. The pigment will appear darker than the final result, as the dye is still on the surface of the skin.

2. **Days 2–3**
   Swelling starts to subside, and the skin around the eyebrows may feel dry or tight.
   The eyebrows will still appear dark, but the skin begins to form a light protective layer.

3. **Days 4–7**
   Exfoliation begins. Scabs may form and fall off naturally, so it's important not to touch, scratch, or try to speed up the process.
   Your eyebrows may look uneven or have „empty" spots, but this is a normal part of healing as the pigment settles.

4. **Days 7–14**
   The scabs gradually fall off, and the pigment may look much lighter. Many people feel that their eyebrows are too light at this stage, but the color will continue to stabilize.
   Continue to avoid excessive washing and using cosmetics on the eyebrow area.

5. **Days 14–21**
   The eyebrows will appear lighter and more natural. Some areas may seem lighter than others, but this is part of the process.
   The pigment begins to settle into the skin, and the final color will start to become more visible.

6. **After 4 Weeks**
   By this point, the eyebrows are fully healed. The color will be 20-50% lighter compared to the first few days post-procedure.
   A touch-up session may be needed to fill any pigment gaps or refine the shape.

Date of your touch-up:

Post-procedure care after micropigmentation

Following a micropigmentation procedure, the skin requires special attention to ensure proper healing and long-lasting, aesthetic results. Below are the recommended post-care instructions:

1. **Hygiene**
   Always wash your hands before touching your eyebrows.
   For the first week, gently cleanse the treated area with lukewarm water.
   Soak a cotton pad in lukewarm water and gently dab your eyebrows, avoiding any rubbing motions.
   Dry the area using a dry cotton pad, again with gentle dabbing to avoid friction.
   Repeat this process 4 times a day at regular intervals.
   For the first two weeks, avoid excessive moisture on the eyebrows (e.g., during baths or showers). After 7-14 days, when the initial healing has occurred, you may begin using a gentle micellar water for cleansing. Avoid products containing alcohol or harsh ingredients.

2. **Preventing Irritation**
   Do not scratch or rub your eyebrows, even if small scabs form. Allow the scabs to fall off naturally to avoid scarring or pigment loss.
   Avoid applying makeup to the eyebrow area until fully healed (approximately 7-14 days).
   For at least 14 days, avoid saunas, swimming pools, hot baths, and excessive sweating, as these can cause the pigment to fade or irritate the skin.

3. **Sun Protection**
   Avoid sun exposure and tanning beds for at least 4 weeks. UV radiation can cause the pigment to fade.
   Once your eyebrows are fully healed, apply a high SPF sunscreen to protect the pigment from fading.

4. **Avoiding Intensive Cosmetic Treatments**
   For 4-6 weeks post-procedure, avoid facial treatments such as chemical peels, laser treatments, or the use of strong creams around the eyebrow area, as these may weaken the pigment.

5. **Consulting a Specialist**
   If you have any concerns or notice unusual symptoms such as excessive redness, swelling, or oozing, contact the cosmetologist who performed the procedure.

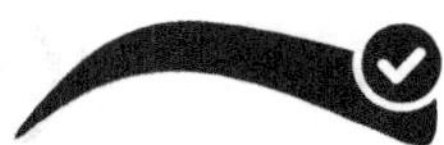

Healing process after micropigmentation

The healing process following permanent eyebrow makeup takes place in several stages and usually lasts between 4 to 6 weeks. During this time, the appearance of your eyebrows will change as the pigment gradually settles into the skin. Below are the stages of the healing process:

1. **Day 1: Immediately After the Procedure**
   Your eyebrows will look very intense, dark, and prominent. The skin may be slightly swollen and red. The pigment will appear darker than the final result, as the dye is still on the surface of the skin.

2. **Days 2–3**
   Swelling starts to subside, and the skin around the eyebrows may feel dry or tight.
   The eyebrows will still appear dark, but the skin begins to form a light protective layer.

3. **Days 4–7**
   Exfoliation begins. Scabs may form and fall off naturally, so it's important not to touch, scratch, or try to speed up the process.
   Your eyebrows may look uneven or have „empty" spots, but this is a normal part of healing as the pigment settles.

4. **Days 7–14**
   The scabs gradually fall off, and the pigment may look much lighter. Many people feel that their eyebrows are too light at this stage, but the color will continue to stabilize.
   Continue to avoid excessive washing and using cosmetics on the eyebrow area.

5. **Days 14–21**
   The eyebrows will appear lighter and more natural. Some areas may seem lighter than others, but this is part of the process.
   The pigment begins to settle into the skin, and the final color will start to become more visible.

6. **After 4 Weeks**
   By this point, the eyebrows are fully healed. The color will be 20-50% lighter compared to the first few days post-procedure.
   A touch-up session may be needed to fill any pigment gaps or refine the shape.

Date of your touch-up:

Post-procedure care after micropigmentation

Following a micropigmentation procedure, the skin requires special attention to ensure proper healing and long-lasting, aesthetic results. Below are the recommended post-care instructions:

① **Hygiene**
Always wash your hands before touching your eyebrows.
For the first week, gently cleanse the treated area with lukewarm water.
Soak a cotton pad in lukewarm water and gently dab your eyebrows, avoiding any rubbing motions.
Dry the area using a dry cotton pad, again with gentle dabbing to avoid friction.
Repeat this process 4 times a day at regular intervals.
For the first two weeks, avoid excessive moisture on the eyebrows (e.g., during baths or showers). After 7-14 days, when the initial healing has occurred, you may begin using a gentle micellar water for cleansing. Avoid products containing alcohol or harsh ingredients.

② **Preventing Irritation**
Do not scratch or rub your eyebrows, even if small scabs form. Allow the scabs to fall off naturally to avoid scarring or pigment loss.
Avoid applying makeup to the eyebrow area until fully healed (approximately 7-14 days).
For at least 14 days, avoid saunas, swimming pools, hot baths, and excessive sweating, as these can cause the pigment to fade or irritate the skin.

③ **Sun Protection**
Avoid sun exposure and tanning beds for at least 4 weeks. UV radiation can cause the pigment to fade.
Once your eyebrows are fully healed, apply a high SPF sunscreen to protect the pigment from fading.

④ **Avoiding Intensive Cosmetic Treatments**
For 4-6 weeks post-procedure, avoid facial treatments such as chemical peels, laser treatments, or the use of strong creams around the eyebrow area, as these may weaken the pigment.

⑤ **Consulting a Specialist**
If you have any concerns or notice unusual symptoms such as excessive redness, swelling, or oozing, contact the cosmetologist who performed the procedure.

Healing process after micropigmentation

The healing process following permanent eyebrow makeup takes place in several stages and usually lasts between 4 to 6 weeks. During this time, the appearance of your eyebrows will change as the pigment gradually settles into the skin. Below are the stages of the healing process:

1. **Day 1: Immediately After the Procedure**
   Your eyebrows will look very intense, dark, and prominent. The skin may be slightly swollen and red. The pigment will appear darker than the final result, as the dye is still on the surface of the skin.

2. **Days 2–3**
   Swelling starts to subside, and the skin around the eyebrows may feel dry or tight.
   The eyebrows will still appear dark, but the skin begins to form a light protective layer.

3. **Days 4–7**
   Exfoliation begins. Scabs may form and fall off naturally, so it's important not to touch, scratch, or try to speed up the process.
   Your eyebrows may look uneven or have „empty" spots, but this is a normal part of healing as the pigment settles.

4. **Days 7–14**
   The scabs gradually fall off, and the pigment may look much lighter. Many people feel that their eyebrows are too light at this stage, but the color will continue to stabilize.
   Continue to avoid excessive washing and using cosmetics on the eyebrow area.

5. **Days 14–21**
   The eyebrows will appear lighter and more natural. Some areas may seem lighter than others, but this is part of the process.
   The pigment begins to settle into the skin, and the final color will start to become more visible.

6. **After 4 Weeks**
   By this point, the eyebrows are fully healed. The color will be 20-50% lighter compared to the first few days post-procedure.
   A touch-up session may be needed to fill any pigment gaps or refine the shape.

Date of your touch-up:

Post-procedure care after micropigmentation

Following a micropigmentation procedure, the skin requires special attention to ensure proper healing and long-lasting, aesthetic results. Below are the recommended post-care instructions:

1. **Hygiene**

   Always wash your hands before touching your eyebrows.

   For the first week, gently cleanse the treated area with lukewarm water.

   Soak a cotton pad in lukewarm water and gently dab your eyebrows, avoiding any rubbing motions.

   Dry the area using a dry cotton pad, again with gentle dabbing to avoid friction.

   Repeat this process 4 times a day at regular intervals.

   For the first two weeks, avoid excessive moisture on the eyebrows (e.g., during baths or showers). After 7-14 days, when the initial healing has occurred, you may begin using a gentle micellar water for cleansing. Avoid products containing alcohol or harsh ingredients.

2. **Preventing Irritation**

   Do not scratch or rub your eyebrows, even if small scabs form. Allow the scabs to fall off naturally to avoid scarring or pigment loss.

   Avoid applying makeup to the eyebrow area until fully healed (approximately 7-14 days).

   For at least 14 days, avoid saunas, swimming pools, hot baths, and excessive sweating, as these can cause the pigment to fade or irritate the skin.

3. **Sun Protection**

   Avoid sun exposure and tanning beds for at least 4 weeks. UV radiation can cause the pigment to fade.

   Once your eyebrows are fully healed, apply a high SPF sunscreen to protect the pigment from fading.

4. **Avoiding Intensive Cosmetic Treatments**

   For 4-6 weeks post-procedure, avoid facial treatments such as chemical peels, laser treatments, or the use of strong creams around the eyebrow area, as these may weaken the pigment.

5. **Consulting a Specialist**

   If you have any concerns or notice unusual symptoms such as excessive redness, swelling, or oozing, contact the cosmetologist who performed the procedure.

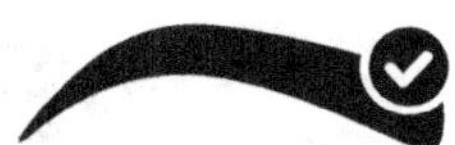

Healing process after micropigmentation

The healing process following permanent eyebrow makeup takes place in several stages and usually lasts between 4 to 6 weeks. During this time, the appearance of your eyebrows will change as the pigment gradually settles into the skin. Below are the stages of the healing process:

① **Day 1: Immediately After the Procedure**
Your eyebrows will look very intense, dark, and prominent. The skin may be slightly swollen and red. The pigment will appear darker than the final result, as the dye is still on the surface of the skin.

② **Days 2–3**
Swelling starts to subside, and the skin around the eyebrows may feel dry or tight.
The eyebrows will still appear dark, but the skin begins to form a light protective layer.

③ **Days 4–7**
Exfoliation begins. Scabs may form and fall off naturally, so it's important not to touch, scratch, or try to speed up the process.
Your eyebrows may look uneven or have „empty" spots, but this is a normal part of healing as the pigment settles.

④ **Days 7–14**
The scabs gradually fall off, and the pigment may look much lighter. Many people feel that their eyebrows are too light at this stage, but the color will continue to stabilize.
Continue to avoid excessive washing and using cosmetics on the eyebrow area.

⑤ **Days 14–21**
The eyebrows will appear lighter and more natural. Some areas may seem lighter than others, but this is part of the process.
The pigment begins to settle into the skin, and the final color will start to become more visible.

⑥ **After 4 Weeks**
By this point, the eyebrows are fully healed. The color will be 20-50% lighter compared to the first few days post-procedure.
A touch-up session may be needed to fill any pigment gaps or refine the shape.

Date of your touch-up:

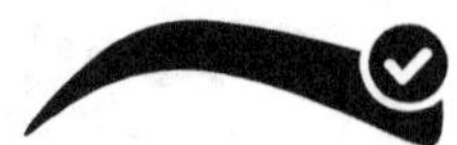

Post-procedure care after micropigmentation

Following a micropigmentation procedure, the skin requires special attention to ensure proper healing and long-lasting, aesthetic results. Below are the recommended post-care instructions:

1. **Hygiene**
   Always wash your hands before touching your eyebrows.
   For the first week, gently cleanse the treated area with lukewarm water.
   Soak a cotton pad in lukewarm water and gently dab your eyebrows, avoiding any rubbing motions.
   Dry the area using a dry cotton pad, again with gentle dabbing to avoid friction.
   Repeat this process 4 times a day at regular intervals.
   For the first two weeks, avoid excessive moisture on the eyebrows (e.g., during baths or showers). After 7-14 days, when the initial healing has occurred, you may begin using a gentle micellar water for cleansing. Avoid products containing alcohol or harsh ingredients.

2. **Preventing Irritation**
   Do not scratch or rub your eyebrows, even if small scabs form. Allow the scabs to fall off naturally to avoid scarring or pigment loss.
   Avoid applying makeup to the eyebrow area until fully healed (approximately 7-14 days).
   For at least 14 days, avoid saunas, swimming pools, hot baths, and excessive sweating, as these can cause the pigment to fade or irritate the skin.

3. **Sun Protection**
   Avoid sun exposure and tanning beds for at least 4 weeks. UV radiation can cause the pigment to fade.
   Once your eyebrows are fully healed, apply a high SPF sunscreen to protect the pigment from fading.

4. **Avoiding Intensive Cosmetic Treatments**
   For 4-6 weeks post-procedure, avoid facial treatments such as chemical peels, laser treatments, or the use of strong creams around the eyebrow area, as these may weaken the pigment.

5. **Consulting a Specialist**
   If you have any concerns or notice unusual symptoms such as excessive redness, swelling, or oozing, contact the cosmetologist who performed the procedure.

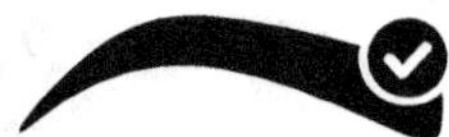

Healing process after micropigmentation

The healing process following permanent eyebrow makeup takes place in several stages and usually lasts between 4 to 6 weeks. During this time, the appearance of your eyebrows will change as the pigment gradually settles into the skin. Below are the stages of the healing process:

1. **Day 1: Immediately After the Procedure**
   Your eyebrows will look very intense, dark, and prominent. The skin may be slightly swollen and red. The pigment will appear darker than the final result, as the dye is still on the surface of the skin.

2. **Days 2–3**
   Swelling starts to subside, and the skin around the eyebrows may feel dry or tight.
   The eyebrows will still appear dark, but the skin begins to form a light protective layer.

3. **Days 4–7**
   Exfoliation begins. Scabs may form and fall off naturally, so it's important not to touch, scratch, or try to speed up the process.
   Your eyebrows may look uneven or have „empty" spots, but this is a normal part of healing as the pigment settles.

4. **Days 7–14**
   The scabs gradually fall off, and the pigment may look much lighter. Many people feel that their eyebrows are too light at this stage, but the color will continue to stabilize.
   Continue to avoid excessive washing and using cosmetics on the eyebrow area.

5. **Days 14–21**
   The eyebrows will appear lighter and more natural. Some areas may seem lighter than others, but this is part of the process.
   The pigment begins to settle into the skin, and the final color will start to become more visible.

6. **After 4 Weeks**
   By this point, the eyebrows are fully healed. The color will be 20-50% lighter compared to the first few days post-procedure.
   A touch-up session may be needed to fill any pigment gaps or refine the shape.

Date of your touch-up:

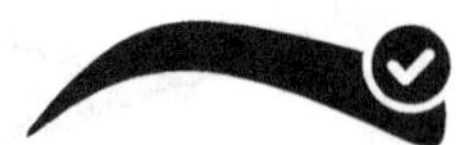

Post-procedure care after micropigmentation

Following a micropigmentation procedure, the skin requires special attention to ensure proper healing and long-lasting, aesthetic results. Below are the recommended post-care instructions:

1. **Hygiene**

   Always wash your hands before touching your eyebrows.
   For the first week, gently cleanse the treated area with lukewarm water.
   Soak a cotton pad in lukewarm water and gently dab your eyebrows, avoiding any rubbing motions.
   Dry the area using a dry cotton pad, again with gentle dabbing to avoid friction.
   Repeat this process 4 times a day at regular intervals.
   For the first two weeks, avoid excessive moisture on the eyebrows (e.g., during baths or showers). After 7-14 days, when the initial healing has occurred, you may begin using a gentle micellar water for cleansing. Avoid products containing alcohol or harsh ingredients.

2. **Preventing Irritation**

   Do not scratch or rub your eyebrows, even if small scabs form. Allow the scabs to fall off naturally to avoid scarring or pigment loss.
   Avoid applying makeup to the eyebrow area until fully healed (approximately 7-14 days).
   For at least 14 days, avoid saunas, swimming pools, hot baths, and excessive sweating, as these can cause the pigment to fade or irritate the skin.

3. **Sun Protection**

   Avoid sun exposure and tanning beds for at least 4 weeks. UV radiation can cause the pigment to fade.
   Once your eyebrows are fully healed, apply a high SPF sunscreen to protect the pigment from fading.

4. **Avoiding Intensive Cosmetic Treatments**

   For 4-6 weeks post-procedure, avoid facial treatments such as chemical peels, laser treatments, or the use of strong creams around the eyebrow area, as these may weaken the pigment.

5. **Consulting a Specialist**

   If you have any concerns or notice unusual symptoms such as excessive redness, swelling, or oozing, contact the cosmetologist who performed the procedure.

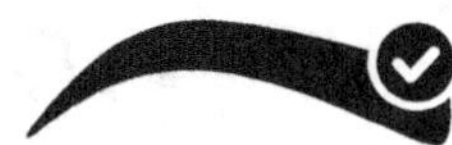

Healing process after micropigmentation

The healing process following permanent eyebrow makeup takes place in several stages and usually lasts between 4 to 6 weeks. During this time, the appearance of your eyebrows will change as the pigment gradually settles into the skin. Below are the stages of the healing process:

① **Day 1: Immediately After the Procedure**
Your eyebrows will look very intense, dark, and prominent. The skin may be slightly swollen and red. The pigment will appear darker than the final result, as the dye is still on the surface of the skin.

② **Days 2–3**
Swelling starts to subside, and the skin around the eyebrows may feel dry or tight.
The eyebrows will still appear dark, but the skin begins to form a light protective layer.

③ **Days 4–7**
Exfoliation begins. Scabs may form and fall off naturally, so it's important not to touch, scratch, or try to speed up the process.
Your eyebrows may look uneven or have „empty" spots, but this is a normal part of healing as the pigment settles.

④ **Days 7–14**
The scabs gradually fall off, and the pigment may look much lighter. Many people feel that their eyebrows are too light at this stage, but the color will continue to stabilize.
Continue to avoid excessive washing and using cosmetics on the eyebrow area.

⑤ **Days 14–21**
The eyebrows will appear lighter and more natural. Some areas may seem lighter than others, but this is part of the process.
The pigment begins to settle into the skin, and the final color will start to become more visible.

⑥ **After 4 Weeks**
By this point, the eyebrows are fully healed. The color will be 20-50% lighter compared to the first few days post-procedure.
A touch-up session may be needed to fill any pigment gaps or refine the shape.

Date of your touch-up:

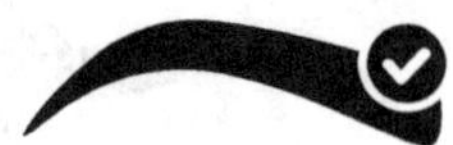

Post-procedure care after micropigmentation

Following a micropigmentation procedure, the skin requires special attention to ensure proper healing and long-lasting, aesthetic results. Below are the recommended post-care instructions:

1. **Hygiene**

   Always wash your hands before touching your eyebrows.

   For the first week, gently cleanse the treated area with lukewarm water.

   Soak a cotton pad in lukewarm water and gently dab your eyebrows, avoiding any rubbing motions.

   Dry the area using a dry cotton pad, again with gentle dabbing to avoid friction.

   Repeat this process 4 times a day at regular intervals.

   For the first two weeks, avoid excessive moisture on the eyebrows (e.g., during baths or showers). After 7-14 days, when the initial healing has occurred, you may begin using a gentle micellar water for cleansing. Avoid products containing alcohol or harsh ingredients.

2. **Preventing Irritation**

   Do not scratch or rub your eyebrows, even if small scabs form. Allow the scabs to fall off naturally to avoid scarring or pigment loss.

   Avoid applying makeup to the eyebrow area until fully healed (approximately 7-14 days).

   For at least 14 days, avoid saunas, swimming pools, hot baths, and excessive sweating, as these can cause the pigment to fade or irritate the skin.

3. **Sun Protection**

   Avoid sun exposure and tanning beds for at least 4 weeks. UV radiation can cause the pigment to fade.

   Once your eyebrows are fully healed, apply a high SPF sunscreen to protect the pigment from fading.

4. **Avoiding Intensive Cosmetic Treatments**

   For 4-6 weeks post-procedure, avoid facial treatments such as chemical peels, laser treatments, or the use of strong creams around the eyebrow area, as these may weaken the pigment.

5. **Consulting a Specialist**

   If you have any concerns or notice unusual symptoms such as excessive redness, swelling, or oozing, contact the cosmetologist who performed the procedure.

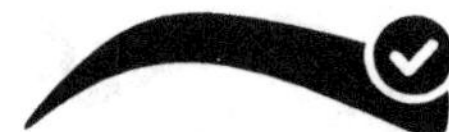

Healing process after micropigmentation

The healing process following permanent eyebrow makeup takes place in several stages and usually lasts between 4 to 6 weeks. During this time, the appearance of your eyebrows will change as the pigment gradually settles into the skin. Below are the stages of the healing process:

1. **Day 1: Immediately After the Procedure**
   Your eyebrows will look very intense, dark, and prominent. The skin may be slightly swollen and red. The pigment will appear darker than the final result, as the dye is still on the surface of the skin.

2. **Days 2–3**
   Swelling starts to subside, and the skin around the eyebrows may feel dry or tight.
   The eyebrows will still appear dark, but the skin begins to form a light protective layer.

3. **Days 4–7**
   Exfoliation begins. Scabs may form and fall off naturally, so it's important not to touch, scratch, or try to speed up the process.
   Your eyebrows may look uneven or have „empty" spots, but this is a normal part of healing as the pigment settles.

4. **Days 7–14**
   The scabs gradually fall off, and the pigment may look much lighter. Many people feel that their eyebrows are too light at this stage, but the color will continue to stabilize.
   Continue to avoid excessive washing and using cosmetics on the eyebrow area.

5. **Days 14–21**
   The eyebrows will appear lighter and more natural. Some areas may seem lighter than others, but this is part of the process.
   The pigment begins to settle into the skin, and the final color will start to become more visible.

6. **After 4 Weeks**
   By this point, the eyebrows are fully healed. The color will be 20-50% lighter compared to the first few days post-procedure.
   A touch-up session may be needed to fill any pigment gaps or refine the shape.

Date of your touch-up:

Post-procedure care after micropigmentation

Following a micropigmentation procedure, the skin requires special attention to ensure proper healing and long-lasting, aesthetic results. Below are the recommended post-care instructions:

1. **Hygiene**
   Always wash your hands before touching your eyebrows.
   For the first week, gently cleanse the treated area with lukewarm water.
   Soak a cotton pad in lukewarm water and gently dab your eyebrows, avoiding any rubbing motions.
   Dry the area using a dry cotton pad, again with gentle dabbing to avoid friction.
   Repeat this process 4 times a day at regular intervals.
   For the first two weeks, avoid excessive moisture on the eyebrows (e.g., during baths or showers). After 7-14 days, when the initial healing has occurred, you may begin using a gentle micellar water for cleansing. Avoid products containing alcohol or harsh ingredients.

2. **Preventing Irritation**
   Do not scratch or rub your eyebrows, even if small scabs form. Allow the scabs to fall off naturally to avoid scarring or pigment loss.
   Avoid applying makeup to the eyebrow area until fully healed (approximately 7-14 days).
   For at least 14 days, avoid saunas, swimming pools, hot baths, and excessive sweating, as these can cause the pigment to fade or irritate the skin.

3. **Sun Protection**
   Avoid sun exposure and tanning beds for at least 4 weeks. UV radiation can cause the pigment to fade.
   Once your eyebrows are fully healed, apply a high SPF sunscreen to protect the pigment from fading.

4. **Avoiding Intensive Cosmetic Treatments**
   For 4-6 weeks post-procedure, avoid facial treatments such as chemical peels, laser treatments, or the use of strong creams around the eyebrow area, as these may weaken the pigment.

5. **Consulting a Specialist**
   If you have any concerns or notice unusual symptoms such as excessive redness, swelling, or oozing, contact the cosmetologist who performed the procedure.

Healing process after micropigmentation

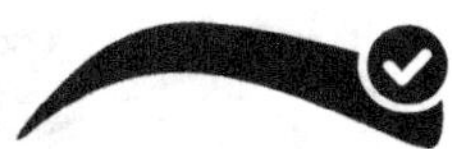

The healing process following permanent eyebrow makeup takes place in several stages and usually lasts between 4 to 6 weeks. During this time, the appearance of your eyebrows will change as the pigment gradually settles into the skin. Below are the stages of the healing process:

1. **Day 1: Immediately After the Procedure**
   Your eyebrows will look very intense, dark, and prominent. The skin may be slightly swollen and red. The pigment will appear darker than the final result, as the dye is still on the surface of the skin.

2. **Days 2–3**
   Swelling starts to subside, and the skin around the eyebrows may feel dry or tight.
   The eyebrows will still appear dark, but the skin begins to form a light protective layer.

3. **Days 4–7**
   Exfoliation begins. Scabs may form and fall off naturally, so it's important not to touch, scratch, or try to speed up the process.
   Your eyebrows may look uneven or have „empty" spots, but this is a normal part of healing as the pigment settles.

4. **Days 7–14**
   The scabs gradually fall off, and the pigment may look much lighter. Many people feel that their eyebrows are too light at this stage, but the color will continue to stabilize.
   Continue to avoid excessive washing and using cosmetics on the eyebrow area.

5. **Days 14–21**
   The eyebrows will appear lighter and more natural. Some areas may seem lighter than others, but this is part of the process.
   The pigment begins to settle into the skin, and the final color will start to become more visible.

6. **After 4 Weeks**
   By this point, the eyebrows are fully healed. The color will be 20-50% lighter compared to the first few days post-procedure.
   A touch-up session may be needed to fill any pigment gaps or refine the shape.

Date of your touch-up:

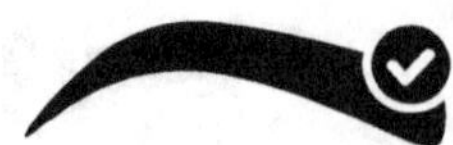

Post-procedure care after micropigmentation

Following a micropigmentation procedure, the skin requires special attention to ensure proper healing and long-lasting, aesthetic results. Below are the recommended post-care instructions:

1. **Hygiene**

   Always wash your hands before touching your eyebrows.

   For the first week, gently cleanse the treated area with lukewarm water.

   Soak a cotton pad in lukewarm water and gently dab your eyebrows, avoiding any rubbing motions.

   Dry the area using a dry cotton pad, again with gentle dabbing to avoid friction.

   Repeat this process 4 times a day at regular intervals.

   For the first two weeks, avoid excessive moisture on the eyebrows (e.g., during baths or showers). After 7-14 days, when the initial healing has occurred, you may begin using a gentle micellar water for cleansing. Avoid products containing alcohol or harsh ingredients.

2. **Preventing Irritation**

   Do not scratch or rub your eyebrows, even if small scabs form. Allow the scabs to fall off naturally to avoid scarring or pigment loss.

   Avoid applying makeup to the eyebrow area until fully healed (approximately 7-14 days).

   For at least 14 days, avoid saunas, swimming pools, hot baths, and excessive sweating, as these can cause the pigment to fade or irritate the skin.

3. **Sun Protection**

   Avoid sun exposure and tanning beds for at least 4 weeks. UV radiation can cause the pigment to fade.

   Once your eyebrows are fully healed, apply a high SPF sunscreen to protect the pigment from fading.

4. **Avoiding Intensive Cosmetic Treatments**

   For 4-6 weeks post-procedure, avoid facial treatments such as chemical peels, laser treatments, or the use of strong creams around the eyebrow area, as these may weaken the pigment.

5. **Consulting a Specialist**

   If you have any concerns or notice unusual symptoms such as excessive redness, swelling, or oozing, contact the cosmetologist who performed the procedure.

Healing process after micropigmentation

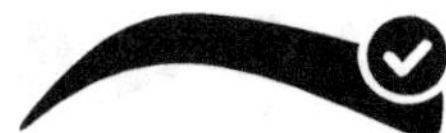

The healing process following permanent eyebrow makeup takes place in several stages and usually lasts between 4 to 6 weeks. During this time, the appearance of your eyebrows will change as the pigment gradually settles into the skin. Below are the stages of the healing process:

1. **Day 1: Immediately After the Procedure**
   Your eyebrows will look very intense, dark, and prominent. The skin may be slightly swollen and red. The pigment will appear darker than the final result, as the dye is still on the surface of the skin.

2. **Days 2–3**
   Swelling starts to subside, and the skin around the eyebrows may feel dry or tight.
   The eyebrows will still appear dark, but the skin begins to form a light protective layer.

3. **Days 4–7**
   Exfoliation begins. Scabs may form and fall off naturally, so it's important not to touch, scratch, or try to speed up the process.
   Your eyebrows may look uneven or have „empty" spots, but this is a normal part of healing as the pigment settles.

4. **Days 7–14**
   The scabs gradually fall off, and the pigment may look much lighter. Many people feel that their eyebrows are too light at this stage, but the color will continue to stabilize.
   Continue to avoid excessive washing and using cosmetics on the eyebrow area.

5. **Days 14–21**
   The eyebrows will appear lighter and more natural. Some areas may seem lighter than others, but this is part of the process.
   The pigment begins to settle into the skin, and the final color will start to become more visible.

6. **After 4 Weeks**
   By this point, the eyebrows are fully healed. The color will be 20-50% lighter compared to the first few days post-procedure.
   A touch-up session may be needed to fill any pigment gaps or refine the shape.

Date of your touch-up:

Post-procedure care after micropigmentation

Following a micropigmentation procedure, the skin requires special attention to ensure proper healing and long-lasting, aesthetic results. Below are the recommended post-care instructions:

1. **Hygiene**

   Always wash your hands before touching your eyebrows.

   For the first week, gently cleanse the treated area with lukewarm water.

   Soak a cotton pad in lukewarm water and gently dab your eyebrows, avoiding any rubbing motions.

   Dry the area using a dry cotton pad, again with gentle dabbing to avoid friction.

   Repeat this process 4 times a day at regular intervals.

   For the first two weeks, avoid excessive moisture on the eyebrows (e.g., during baths or showers). After 7-14 days, when the initial healing has occurred, you may begin using a gentle micellar water for cleansing. Avoid products containing alcohol or harsh ingredients.

2. **Preventing Irritation**

   Do not scratch or rub your eyebrows, even if small scabs form. Allow the scabs to fall off naturally to avoid scarring or pigment loss.

   Avoid applying makeup to the eyebrow area until fully healed (approximately 7-14 days).

   For at least 14 days, avoid saunas, swimming pools, hot baths, and excessive sweating, as these can cause the pigment to fade or irritate the skin.

3. **Sun Protection**

   Avoid sun exposure and tanning beds for at least 4 weeks. UV radiation can cause the pigment to fade.

   Once your eyebrows are fully healed, apply a high SPF sunscreen to protect the pigment from fading.

4. **Avoiding Intensive Cosmetic Treatments**

   For 4-6 weeks post-procedure, avoid facial treatments such as chemical peels, laser treatments, or the use of strong creams around the eyebrow area, as these may weaken the pigment.

5. **Consulting a Specialist**

   If you have any concerns or notice unusual symptoms such as excessive redness, swelling, or oozing, contact the cosmetologist who performed the procedure.

Healing process after micropigmentation

The healing process following permanent eyebrow makeup takes place in several stages and usually lasts between 4 to 6 weeks. During this time, the appearance of your eyebrows will change as the pigment gradually settles into the skin. Below are the stages of the healing process:

1. **Day 1: Immediately After the Procedure**
   Your eyebrows will look very intense, dark, and prominent. The skin may be slightly swollen and red. The pigment will appear darker than the final result, as the dye is still on the surface of the skin.

2. **Days 2–3**
   Swelling starts to subside, and the skin around the eyebrows may feel dry or tight.
   The eyebrows will still appear dark, but the skin begins to form a light protective layer.

3. **Days 4–7**
   Exfoliation begins. Scabs may form and fall off naturally, so it's important not to touch, scratch, or try to speed up the process.
   Your eyebrows may look uneven or have „empty" spots, but this is a normal part of healing as the pigment settles.

4. **Days 7–14**
   The scabs gradually fall off, and the pigment may look much lighter. Many people feel that their eyebrows are too light at this stage, but the color will continue to stabilize.
   Continue to avoid excessive washing and using cosmetics on the eyebrow area.

5. **Days 14–21**
   The eyebrows will appear lighter and more natural. Some areas may seem lighter than others, but this is part of the process.
   The pigment begins to settle into the skin, and the final color will start to become more visible.

6. **After 4 Weeks**
   By this point, the eyebrows are fully healed. The color will be 20-50% lighter compared to the first few days post-procedure.
   A touch-up session may be needed to fill any pigment gaps or refine the shape.

Date of your touch-up:

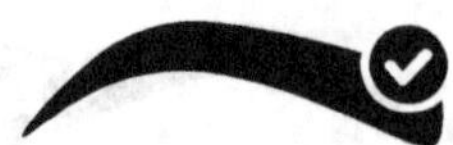

Post-procedure care after micropigmentation

Following a micropigmentation procedure, the skin requires special attention to ensure proper healing and long-lasting, aesthetic results. Below are the recommended post-care instructions:

1. **Hygiene**
   Always wash your hands before touching your eyebrows.
   For the first week, gently cleanse the treated area with lukewarm water.
   Soak a cotton pad in lukewarm water and gently dab your eyebrows, avoiding any rubbing motions.
   Dry the area using a dry cotton pad, again with gentle dabbing to avoid friction.
   Repeat this process 4 times a day at regular intervals.
   For the first two weeks, avoid excessive moisture on the eyebrows (e.g., during baths or showers). After 7-14 days, when the initial healing has occurred, you may begin using a gentle micellar water for cleansing. Avoid products containing alcohol or harsh ingredients.

2. **Preventing Irritation**
   Do not scratch or rub your eyebrows, even if small scabs form. Allow the scabs to fall off naturally to avoid scarring or pigment loss.
   Avoid applying makeup to the eyebrow area until fully healed (approximately 7-14 days).
   For at least 14 days, avoid saunas, swimming pools, hot baths, and excessive sweating, as these can cause the pigment to fade or irritate the skin.

3. **Sun Protection**
   Avoid sun exposure and tanning beds for at least 4 weeks. UV radiation can cause the pigment to fade.
   Once your eyebrows are fully healed, apply a high SPF sunscreen to protect the pigment from fading.

4. **Avoiding Intensive Cosmetic Treatments**
   For 4-6 weeks post-procedure, avoid facial treatments such as chemical peels, laser treatments, or the use of strong creams around the eyebrow area, as these may weaken the pigment.

5. **Consulting a Specialist**
   If you have any concerns or notice unusual symptoms such as excessive redness, swelling, or oozing, contact the cosmetologist who performed the procedure.

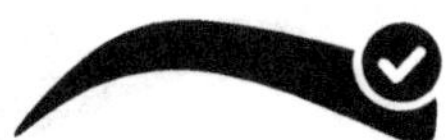

Healing process after micropigmentation

The healing process following permanent eyebrow makeup takes place in several stages and usually lasts between 4 to 6 weeks. During this time, the appearance of your eyebrows will change as the pigment gradually settles into the skin. Below are the stages of the healing process:

① **Day 1: Immediately After the Procedure**
Your eyebrows will look very intense, dark, and prominent. The skin may be slightly swollen and red. The pigment will appear darker than the final result, as the dye is still on the surface of the skin.

② **Days 2–3**
Swelling starts to subside, and the skin around the eyebrows may feel dry or tight.
The eyebrows will still appear dark, but the skin begins to form a light protective layer.

③ **Days 4–7**
Exfoliation begins. Scabs may form and fall off naturally, so it's important not to touch, scratch, or try to speed up the process.
Your eyebrows may look uneven or have „empty" spots, but this is a normal part of healing as the pigment settles.

④ **Days 7–14**
The scabs gradually fall off, and the pigment may look much lighter. Many people feel that their eyebrows are too light at this stage, but the color will continue to stabilize.
Continue to avoid excessive washing and using cosmetics on the eyebrow area.

⑤ **Days 14–21**
The eyebrows will appear lighter and more natural. Some areas may seem lighter than others, but this is part of the process.
The pigment begins to settle into the skin, and the final color will start to become more visible.

⑥ **After 4 Weeks**
By this point, the eyebrows are fully healed. The color will be 20-50% lighter compared to the first few days post-procedure.
A touch-up session may be needed to fill any pigment gaps or refine the shape.

Date of your touch-up:

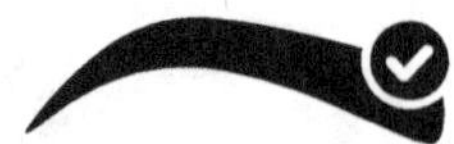

Post-procedure care after micropigmentation

Following a micropigmentation procedure, the skin requires special attention to ensure proper healing and long-lasting, aesthetic results. Below are the recommended post-care instructions:

1. **Hygiene**

   Always wash your hands before touching your eyebrows.

   For the first week, gently cleanse the treated area with lukewarm water.

   Soak a cotton pad in lukewarm water and gently dab your eyebrows, avoiding any rubbing motions.

   Dry the area using a dry cotton pad, again with gentle dabbing to avoid friction.

   Repeat this process 4 times a day at regular intervals.

   For the first two weeks, avoid excessive moisture on the eyebrows (e.g., during baths or showers). After 7-14 days, when the initial healing has occurred, you may begin using a gentle micellar water for cleansing. Avoid products containing alcohol or harsh ingredients.

2. **Preventing Irritation**

   Do not scratch or rub your eyebrows, even if small scabs form. Allow the scabs to fall off naturally to avoid scarring or pigment loss.

   Avoid applying makeup to the eyebrow area until fully healed (approximately 7-14 days).

   For at least 14 days, avoid saunas, swimming pools, hot baths, and excessive sweating, as these can cause the pigment to fade or irritate the skin.

3. **Sun Protection**

   Avoid sun exposure and tanning beds for at least 4 weeks. UV radiation can cause the pigment to fade.

   Once your eyebrows are fully healed, apply a high SPF sunscreen to protect the pigment from fading.

4. **Avoiding Intensive Cosmetic Treatments**

   For 4-6 weeks post-procedure, avoid facial treatments such as chemical peels, laser treatments, or the use of strong creams around the eyebrow area, as these may weaken the pigment.

5. **Consulting a Specialist**

   If you have any concerns or notice unusual symptoms such as excessive redness, swelling, or oozing, contact the cosmetologist who performed the procedure.

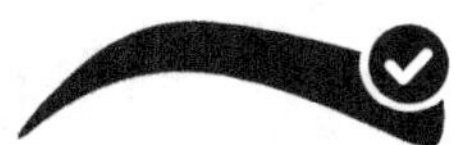

Healing process after micropigmentation

The healing process following permanent eyebrow makeup takes place in several stages and usually lasts between 4 to 6 weeks. During this time, the appearance of your eyebrows will change as the pigment gradually settles into the skin. Below are the stages of the healing process:

1. **Day 1: Immediately After the Procedure**
   Your eyebrows will look very intense, dark, and prominent. The skin may be slightly swollen and red. The pigment will appear darker than the final result, as the dye is still on the surface of the skin.

2. **Days 2–3**
   Swelling starts to subside, and the skin around the eyebrows may feel dry or tight.
   The eyebrows will still appear dark, but the skin begins to form a light protective layer.

3. **Days 4–7**
   Exfoliation begins. Scabs may form and fall off naturally, so it's important not to touch, scratch, or try to speed up the process.
   Your eyebrows may look uneven or have „empty" spots, but this is a normal part of healing as the pigment settles.

4. **Days 7–14**
   The scabs gradually fall off, and the pigment may look much lighter. Many people feel that their eyebrows are too light at this stage, but the color will continue to stabilize.
   Continue to avoid excessive washing and using cosmetics on the eyebrow area.

5. **Days 14–21**
   The eyebrows will appear lighter and more natural. Some areas may seem lighter than others, but this is part of the process.
   The pigment begins to settle into the skin, and the final color will start to become more visible.

6. **After 4 Weeks**
   By this point, the eyebrows are fully healed. The color will be 20-50% lighter compared to the first few days post-procedure.
   A touch-up session may be needed to fill any pigment gaps or refine the shape.

Date of your touch-up:

Post-procedure care after micropigmentation

Following a micropigmentation procedure, the skin requires special attention to ensure proper healing and long-lasting, aesthetic results. Below are the recommended post-care instructions:

1. **Hygiene**
   Always wash your hands before touching your eyebrows.
   For the first week, gently cleanse the treated area with lukewarm water.
   Soak a cotton pad in lukewarm water and gently dab your eyebrows, avoiding any rubbing motions.
   Dry the area using a dry cotton pad, again with gentle dabbing to avoid friction.
   Repeat this process 4 times a day at regular intervals.
   For the first two weeks, avoid excessive moisture on the eyebrows (e.g., during baths or showers). After 7-14 days, when the initial healing has occurred, you may begin using a gentle micellar water for cleansing. Avoid products containing alcohol or harsh ingredients.

2. **Preventing Irritation**
   Do not scratch or rub your eyebrows, even if small scabs form. Allow the scabs to fall off naturally to avoid scarring or pigment loss.
   Avoid applying makeup to the eyebrow area until fully healed (approximately 7-14 days).
   For at least 14 days, avoid saunas, swimming pools, hot baths, and excessive sweating, as these can cause the pigment to fade or irritate the skin.

3. **Sun Protection**
   Avoid sun exposure and tanning beds for at least 4 weeks. UV radiation can cause the pigment to fade.
   Once your eyebrows are fully healed, apply a high SPF sunscreen to protect the pigment from fading.

4. **Avoiding Intensive Cosmetic Treatments**
   For 4-6 weeks post-procedure, avoid facial treatments such as chemical peels, laser treatments, or the use of strong creams around the eyebrow area, as these may weaken the pigment.

5. **Consulting a Specialist**
   If you have any concerns or notice unusual symptoms such as excessive redness, swelling, or oozing, contact the cosmetologist who performed the procedure.

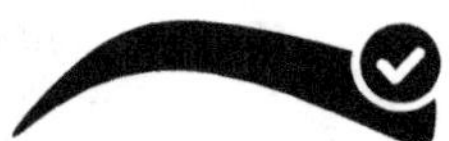

Healing process after micropigmentation

The healing process following permanent eyebrow makeup takes place in several stages and usually lasts between 4 to 6 weeks. During this time, the appearance of your eyebrows will change as the pigment gradually settles into the skin. Below are the stages of the healing process:

(1) **Day 1: Immediately After the Procedure**

Your eyebrows will look very intense, dark, and prominent. The skin may be slightly swollen and red. The pigment will appear darker than the final result, as the dye is still on the surface of the skin.

(2) **Days 2–3**

Swelling starts to subside, and the skin around the eyebrows may feel dry or tight.
The eyebrows will still appear dark, but the skin begins to form a light protective layer.

(3) **Days 4–7**

Exfoliation begins. Scabs may form and fall off naturally, so it's important not to touch, scratch, or try to speed up the process.
Your eyebrows may look uneven or have „empty" spots, but this is a normal part of healing as the pigment settles.

(4) **Days 7–14**

The scabs gradually fall off, and the pigment may look much lighter. Many people feel that their eyebrows are too light at this stage, but the color will continue to stabilize.
Continue to avoid excessive washing and using cosmetics on the eyebrow area.

(5) **Days 14–21**

The eyebrows will appear lighter and more natural. Some areas may seem lighter than others, but this is part of the process.
The pigment begins to settle into the skin, and the final color will start to become more visible.

(6) **After 4 Weeks**

By this point, the eyebrows are fully healed. The color will be 20-50% lighter compared to the first few days post-procedure.
A touch-up session may be needed to fill any pigment gaps or refine the shape.

Date of your touch-up:

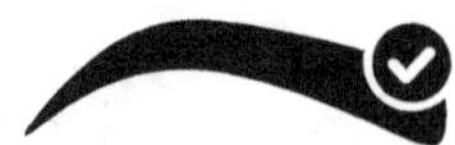

Post-procedure care after micropigmentation

Following a micropigmentation procedure, the skin requires special attention to ensure proper healing and long-lasting, aesthetic results. Below are the recommended post-care instructions:

1. **Hygiene**

   Always wash your hands before touching your eyebrows.

   For the first week, gently cleanse the treated area with lukewarm water.

   Soak a cotton pad in lukewarm water and gently dab your eyebrows, avoiding any rubbing motions.

   Dry the area using a dry cotton pad, again with gentle dabbing to avoid friction.

   Repeat this process 4 times a day at regular intervals.

   For the first two weeks, avoid excessive moisture on the eyebrows (e.g., during baths or showers). After 7-14 days, when the initial healing has occurred, you may begin using a gentle micellar water for cleansing. Avoid products containing alcohol or harsh ingredients.

2. **Preventing Irritation**

   Do not scratch or rub your eyebrows, even if small scabs form. Allow the scabs to fall off naturally to avoid scarring or pigment loss.

   Avoid applying makeup to the eyebrow area until fully healed (approximately 7-14 days).

   For at least 14 days, avoid saunas, swimming pools, hot baths, and excessive sweating, as these can cause the pigment to fade or irritate the skin.

3. **Sun Protection**

   Avoid sun exposure and tanning beds for at least 4 weeks. UV radiation can cause the pigment to fade.

   Once your eyebrows are fully healed, apply a high SPF sunscreen to protect the pigment from fading.

4. **Avoiding Intensive Cosmetic Treatments**

   For 4-6 weeks post-procedure, avoid facial treatments such as chemical peels, laser treatments, or the use of strong creams around the eyebrow area, as these may weaken the pigment.

5. **Consulting a Specialist**

   If you have any concerns or notice unusual symptoms such as excessive redness, swelling, or oozing, contact the cosmetologist who performed the procedure.

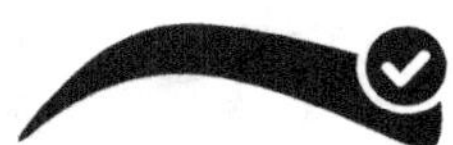

Healing process after micropigmentation

The healing process following permanent eyebrow makeup takes place in several stages and usually lasts between 4 to 6 weeks. During this time, the appearance of your eyebrows will change as the pigment gradually settles into the skin. Below are the stages of the healing process:

1. **Day 1: Immediately After the Procedure**
   Your eyebrows will look very intense, dark, and prominent. The skin may be slightly swollen and red. The pigment will appear darker than the final result, as the dye is still on the surface of the skin.

2. **Days 2–3**
   Swelling starts to subside, and the skin around the eyebrows may feel dry or tight.
   The eyebrows will still appear dark, but the skin begins to form a light protective layer.

3. **Days 4–7**
   Exfoliation begins. Scabs may form and fall off naturally, so it's important not to touch, scratch, or try to speed up the process.
   Your eyebrows may look uneven or have „empty" spots, but this is a normal part of healing as the pigment settles.

4. **Days 7–14**
   The scabs gradually fall off, and the pigment may look much lighter. Many people feel that their eyebrows are too light at this stage, but the color will continue to stabilize.
   Continue to avoid excessive washing and using cosmetics on the eyebrow area.

5. **Days 14–21**
   The eyebrows will appear lighter and more natural. Some areas may seem lighter than others, but this is part of the process.
   The pigment begins to settle into the skin, and the final color will start to become more visible.

6. **After 4 Weeks**
   By this point, the eyebrows are fully healed. The color will be 20-50% lighter compared to the first few days post-procedure.
   A touch-up session may be needed to fill any pigment gaps or refine the shape.

Date of your touch-up:

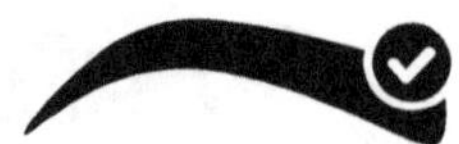

Post-procedure care after micropigmentation

Following a micropigmentation procedure, the skin requires special attention to ensure proper healing and long-lasting, aesthetic results. Below are the recommended post-care instructions:

1. **Hygiene**

   Always wash your hands before touching your eyebrows.

   For the first week, gently cleanse the treated area with lukewarm water.

   Soak a cotton pad in lukewarm water and gently dab your eyebrows, avoiding any rubbing motions.

   Dry the area using a dry cotton pad, again with gentle dabbing to avoid friction.

   Repeat this process 4 times a day at regular intervals.

   For the first two weeks, avoid excessive moisture on the eyebrows (e.g., during baths or showers). After 7-14 days, when the initial healing has occurred, you may begin using a gentle micellar water for cleansing. Avoid products containing alcohol or harsh ingredients.

2. **Preventing Irritation**

   Do not scratch or rub your eyebrows, even if small scabs form. Allow the scabs to fall off naturally to avoid scarring or pigment loss.

   Avoid applying makeup to the eyebrow area until fully healed (approximately 7-14 days).

   For at least 14 days, avoid saunas, swimming pools, hot baths, and excessive sweating, as these can cause the pigment to fade or irritate the skin.

3. **Sun Protection**

   Avoid sun exposure and tanning beds for at least 4 weeks. UV radiation can cause the pigment to fade.

   Once your eyebrows are fully healed, apply a high SPF sunscreen to protect the pigment from fading.

4. **Avoiding Intensive Cosmetic Treatments**

   For 4-6 weeks post-procedure, avoid facial treatments such as chemical peels, laser treatments, or the use of strong creams around the eyebrow area, as these may weaken the pigment.

5. **Consulting a Specialist**

   If you have any concerns or notice unusual symptoms such as excessive redness, swelling, or oozing, contact the cosmetologist who performed the procedure.

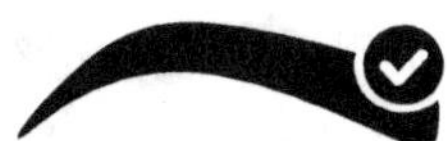

Healing process after micropigmentation

The healing process following permanent eyebrow makeup takes place in several stages and usually lasts between 4 to 6 weeks. During this time, the appearance of your eyebrows will change as the pigment gradually settles into the skin. Below are the stages of the healing process:

1. **Day 1: Immediately After the Procedure**
   Your eyebrows will look very intense, dark, and prominent. The skin may be slightly swollen and red. The pigment will appear darker than the final result, as the dye is still on the surface of the skin.

2. **Days 2–3**
   Swelling starts to subside, and the skin around the eyebrows may feel dry or tight.
   The eyebrows will still appear dark, but the skin begins to form a light protective layer.

3. **Days 4–7**
   Exfoliation begins. Scabs may form and fall off naturally, so it's important not to touch, scratch, or try to speed up the process.
   Your eyebrows may look uneven or have „empty" spots, but this is a normal part of healing as the pigment settles.

4. **Days 7–14**
   The scabs gradually fall off, and the pigment may look much lighter. Many people feel that their eyebrows are too light at this stage, but the color will continue to stabilize.
   Continue to avoid excessive washing and using cosmetics on the eyebrow area.

5. **Days 14–21**
   The eyebrows will appear lighter and more natural. Some areas may seem lighter than others, but this is part of the process.
   The pigment begins to settle into the skin, and the final color will start to become more visible.

6. **After 4 Weeks**
   By this point, the eyebrows are fully healed. The color will be 20-50% lighter compared to the first few days post-procedure.
   A touch-up session may be needed to fill any pigment gaps or refine the shape.

Date of your touch-up:

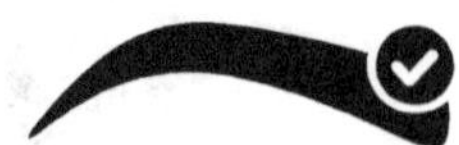

Post-procedure care after micropigmentation

Following a micropigmentation procedure, the skin requires special attention to ensure proper healing and long-lasting, aesthetic results. Below are the recommended post-care instructions:

1. **Hygiene**

   Always wash your hands before touching your eyebrows.

   For the first week, gently cleanse the treated area with lukewarm water.

   Soak a cotton pad in lukewarm water and gently dab your eyebrows, avoiding any rubbing motions.

   Dry the area using a dry cotton pad, again with gentle dabbing to avoid friction.

   Repeat this process 4 times a day at regular intervals.

   For the first two weeks, avoid excessive moisture on the eyebrows (e.g., during baths or showers). After 7-14 days, when the initial healing has occurred, you may begin using a gentle micellar water for cleansing. Avoid products containing alcohol or harsh ingredients.

2. **Preventing Irritation**

   Do not scratch or rub your eyebrows, even if small scabs form. Allow the scabs to fall off naturally to avoid scarring or pigment loss.

   Avoid applying makeup to the eyebrow area until fully healed (approximately 7-14 days).

   For at least 14 days, avoid saunas, swimming pools, hot baths, and excessive sweating, as these can cause the pigment to fade or irritate the skin.

3. **Sun Protection**

   Avoid sun exposure and tanning beds for at least 4 weeks. UV radiation can cause the pigment to fade.

   Once your eyebrows are fully healed, apply a high SPF sunscreen to protect the pigment from fading.

4. **Avoiding Intensive Cosmetic Treatments**

   For 4-6 weeks post-procedure, avoid facial treatments such as chemical peels, laser treatments, or the use of strong creams around the eyebrow area, as these may weaken the pigment.

5. **Consulting a Specialist**

   If you have any concerns or notice unusual symptoms such as excessive redness, swelling, or oozing, contact the cosmetologist who performed the procedure.

Healing process after micropigmentation

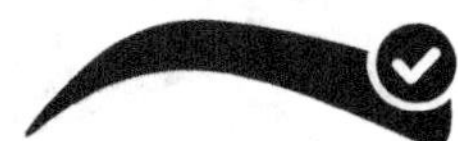

The healing process following permanent eyebrow makeup takes place in several stages and usually lasts between 4 to 6 weeks. During this time, the appearance of your eyebrows will change as the pigment gradually settles into the skin. Below are the stages of the healing process:

1. **Day 1: Immediately After the Procedure**
   Your eyebrows will look very intense, dark, and prominent. The skin may be slightly swollen and red. The pigment will appear darker than the final result, as the dye is still on the surface of the skin.

2. **Days 2–3**
   Swelling starts to subside, and the skin around the eyebrows may feel dry or tight.
   The eyebrows will still appear dark, but the skin begins to form a light protective layer.

3. **Days 4–7**
   Exfoliation begins. Scabs may form and fall off naturally, so it's important not to touch, scratch, or try to speed up the process.
   Your eyebrows may look uneven or have „empty" spots, but this is a normal part of healing as the pigment settles.

4. **Days 7–14**
   The scabs gradually fall off, and the pigment may look much lighter. Many people feel that their eyebrows are too light at this stage, but the color will continue to stabilize.
   Continue to avoid excessive washing and using cosmetics on the eyebrow area.

5. **Days 14–21**
   The eyebrows will appear lighter and more natural. Some areas may seem lighter than others, but this is part of the process.
   The pigment begins to settle into the skin, and the final color will start to become more visible.

6. **After 4 Weeks**
   By this point, the eyebrows are fully healed. The color will be 20-50% lighter compared to the first few days post-procedure.
   A touch-up session may be needed to fill any pigment gaps or refine the shape.

Date of your touch-up:

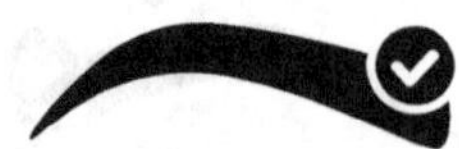

Post-procedure care after micropigmentation

Following a micropigmentation procedure, the skin requires special attention to ensure proper healing and long-lasting, aesthetic results. Below are the recommended post-care instructions:

1. **Hygiene**

   Always wash your hands before touching your eyebrows.

   For the first week, gently cleanse the treated area with lukewarm water.

   Soak a cotton pad in lukewarm water and gently dab your eyebrows, avoiding any rubbing motions.

   Dry the area using a dry cotton pad, again with gentle dabbing to avoid friction.

   Repeat this process 4 times a day at regular intervals.

   For the first two weeks, avoid excessive moisture on the eyebrows (e.g., during baths or showers). After 7-14 days, when the initial healing has occurred, you may begin using a gentle micellar water for cleansing. Avoid products containing alcohol or harsh ingredients.

2. **Preventing Irritation**

   Do not scratch or rub your eyebrows, even if small scabs form. Allow the scabs to fall off naturally to avoid scarring or pigment loss.

   Avoid applying makeup to the eyebrow area until fully healed (approximately 7-14 days).

   For at least 14 days, avoid saunas, swimming pools, hot baths, and excessive sweating, as these can cause the pigment to fade or irritate the skin.

3. **Sun Protection**

   Avoid sun exposure and tanning beds for at least 4 weeks. UV radiation can cause the pigment to fade.

   Once your eyebrows are fully healed, apply a high SPF sunscreen to protect the pigment from fading.

4. **Avoiding Intensive Cosmetic Treatments**

   For 4-6 weeks post-procedure, avoid facial treatments such as chemical peels, laser treatments, or the use of strong creams around the eyebrow area, as these may weaken the pigment.

5. **Consulting a Specialist**

   If you have any concerns or notice unusual symptoms such as excessive redness, swelling, or oozing, contact the cosmetologist who performed the procedure.

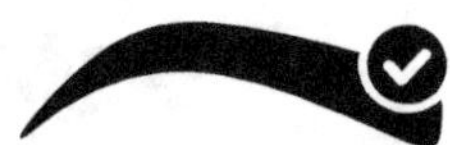

Healing process after micropigmentation

The healing process following permanent eyebrow makeup takes place in several stages and usually lasts between 4 to 6 weeks. During this time, the appearance of your eyebrows will change as the pigment gradually settles into the skin. Below are the stages of the healing process:

1. **Day 1: Immediately After the Procedure**
   Your eyebrows will look very intense, dark, and prominent. The skin may be slightly swollen and red. The pigment will appear darker than the final result, as the dye is still on the surface of the skin.

2. **Days 2–3**
   Swelling starts to subside, and the skin around the eyebrows may feel dry or tight.
   The eyebrows will still appear dark, but the skin begins to form a light protective layer.

3. **Days 4–7**
   Exfoliation begins. Scabs may form and fall off naturally, so it's important not to touch, scratch, or try to speed up the process.
   Your eyebrows may look uneven or have „empty" spots, but this is a normal part of healing as the pigment settles.

4. **Days 7–14**
   The scabs gradually fall off, and the pigment may look much lighter. Many people feel that their eyebrows are too light at this stage, but the color will continue to stabilize.
   Continue to avoid excessive washing and using cosmetics on the eyebrow area.

5. **Days 14–21**
   The eyebrows will appear lighter and more natural. Some areas may seem lighter than others, but this is part of the process.
   The pigment begins to settle into the skin, and the final color will start to become more visible.

6. **After 4 Weeks**
   By this point, the eyebrows are fully healed. The color will be 20-50% lighter compared to the first few days post-procedure.
   A touch-up session may be needed to fill any pigment gaps or refine the shape.

Date of your touch-up:

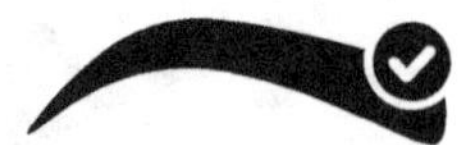

Post-procedure care after micropigmentation

Following a micropigmentation procedure, the skin requires special attention to ensure proper healing and long-lasting, aesthetic results. Below are the recommended post-care instructions:

1. **Hygiene**
   Always wash your hands before touching your eyebrows.
   For the first week, gently cleanse the treated area with lukewarm water.
   Soak a cotton pad in lukewarm water and gently dab your eyebrows, avoiding any rubbing motions.
   Dry the area using a dry cotton pad, again with gentle dabbing to avoid friction.
   Repeat this process 4 times a day at regular intervals.
   For the first two weeks, avoid excessive moisture on the eyebrows (e.g., during baths or showers). After 7-14 days, when the initial healing has occurred, you may begin using a gentle micellar water for cleansing. Avoid products containing alcohol or harsh ingredients.

2. **Preventing Irritation**
   Do not scratch or rub your eyebrows, even if small scabs form. Allow the scabs to fall off naturally to avoid scarring or pigment loss.
   Avoid applying makeup to the eyebrow area until fully healed (approximately 7-14 days).
   For at least 14 days, avoid saunas, swimming pools, hot baths, and excessive sweating, as these can cause the pigment to fade or irritate the skin.

3. **Sun Protection**
   Avoid sun exposure and tanning beds for at least 4 weeks. UV radiation can cause the pigment to fade.
   Once your eyebrows are fully healed, apply a high SPF sunscreen to protect the pigment from fading.

4. **Avoiding Intensive Cosmetic Treatments**
   For 4-6 weeks post-procedure, avoid facial treatments such as chemical peels, laser treatments, or the use of strong creams around the eyebrow area, as these may weaken the pigment.

5. **Consulting a Specialist**
   If you have any concerns or notice unusual symptoms such as excessive redness, swelling, or oozing, contact the cosmetologist who performed the procedure.

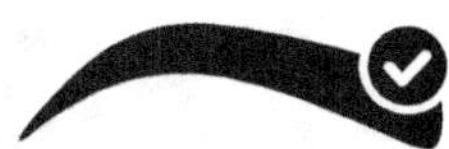

Healing process after micropigmentation

The healing process following permanent eyebrow makeup takes place in several stages and usually lasts between 4 to 6 weeks. During this time, the appearance of your eyebrows will change as the pigment gradually settles into the skin. Below are the stages of the healing process:

1. **Day 1: Immediately After the Procedure**
   Your eyebrows will look very intense, dark, and prominent. The skin may be slightly swollen and red. The pigment will appear darker than the final result, as the dye is still on the surface of the skin.

2. **Days 2–3**
   Swelling starts to subside, and the skin around the eyebrows may feel dry or tight.
   The eyebrows will still appear dark, but the skin begins to form a light protective layer.

3. **Days 4–7**
   Exfoliation begins. Scabs may form and fall off naturally, so it's important not to touch, scratch, or try to speed up the process.
   Your eyebrows may look uneven or have „empty" spots, but this is a normal part of healing as the pigment settles.

4. **Days 7–14**
   The scabs gradually fall off, and the pigment may look much lighter. Many people feel that their eyebrows are too light at this stage, but the color will continue to stabilize.
   Continue to avoid excessive washing and using cosmetics on the eyebrow area.

5. **Days 14–21**
   The eyebrows will appear lighter and more natural. Some areas may seem lighter than others, but this is part of the process.
   The pigment begins to settle into the skin, and the final color will start to become more visible.

6. **After 4 Weeks**
   By this point, the eyebrows are fully healed. The color will be 20-50% lighter compared to the first few days post-procedure.
   A touch-up session may be needed to fill any pigment gaps or refine the shape.

Date of your touch-up:

Post-procedure care after micropigmentation

Following a micropigmentation procedure, the skin requires special attention to ensure proper healing and long-lasting, aesthetic results. Below are the recommended post-care instructions:

1. **Hygiene**
   Always wash your hands before touching your eyebrows.
   For the first week, gently cleanse the treated area with lukewarm water.
   Soak a cotton pad in lukewarm water and gently dab your eyebrows, avoiding any rubbing motions.
   Dry the area using a dry cotton pad, again with gentle dabbing to avoid friction.
   Repeat this process 4 times a day at regular intervals.
   For the first two weeks, avoid excessive moisture on the eyebrows (e.g., during baths or showers). After 7-14 days, when the initial healing has occurred, you may begin using a gentle micellar water for cleansing. Avoid products containing alcohol or harsh ingredients.

2. **Preventing Irritation**
   Do not scratch or rub your eyebrows, even if small scabs form. Allow the scabs to fall off naturally to avoid scarring or pigment loss.
   Avoid applying makeup to the eyebrow area until fully healed (approximately 7-14 days).
   For at least 14 days, avoid saunas, swimming pools, hot baths, and excessive sweating, as these can cause the pigment to fade or irritate the skin.

3. **Sun Protection**
   Avoid sun exposure and tanning beds for at least 4 weeks. UV radiation can cause the pigment to fade.
   Once your eyebrows are fully healed, apply a high SPF sunscreen to protect the pigment from fading.

4. **Avoiding Intensive Cosmetic Treatments**
   For 4-6 weeks post-procedure, avoid facial treatments such as chemical peels, laser treatments, or the use of strong creams around the eyebrow area, as these may weaken the pigment.

5. **Consulting a Specialist**
   If you have any concerns or notice unusual symptoms such as excessive redness, swelling, or oozing, contact the cosmetologist who performed the procedure.

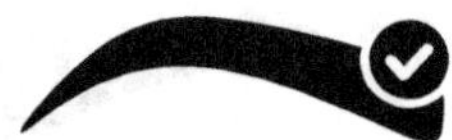

Healing process after micropigmentation

The healing process following permanent eyebrow makeup takes place in several stages and usually lasts between 4 to 6 weeks. During this time, the appearance of your eyebrows will change as the pigment gradually settles into the skin. Below are the stages of the healing process:

1. **Day 1: Immediately After the Procedure**

   Your eyebrows will look very intense, dark, and prominent. The skin may be slightly swollen and red. The pigment will appear darker than the final result, as the dye is still on the surface of the skin.

2. **Days 2–3**

   Swelling starts to subside, and the skin around the eyebrows may feel dry or tight.
   The eyebrows will still appear dark, but the skin begins to form a light protective layer.

3. **Days 4–7**

   Exfoliation begins. Scabs may form and fall off naturally, so it's important not to touch, scratch, or try to speed up the process.
   Your eyebrows may look uneven or have „empty" spots, but this is a normal part of healing as the pigment settles.

4. **Days 7–14**

   The scabs gradually fall off, and the pigment may look much lighter. Many people feel that their eyebrows are too light at this stage, but the color will continue to stabilize.
   Continue to avoid excessive washing and using cosmetics on the eyebrow area.

5. **Days 14–21**

   The eyebrows will appear lighter and more natural. Some areas may seem lighter than others, but this is part of the process.
   The pigment begins to settle into the skin, and the final color will start to become more visible.

6. **After 4 Weeks**

   By this point, the eyebrows are fully healed. The color will be 20-50% lighter compared to the first few days post-procedure.
   A touch-up session may be needed to fill any pigment gaps or refine the shape.

Date of your touch-up:

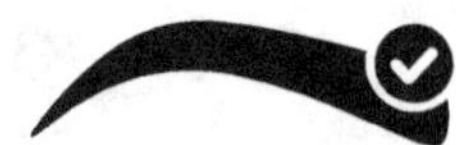

Post-procedure care after micropigmentation

Following a micropigmentation procedure, the skin requires special attention to ensure proper healing and long-lasting, aesthetic results. Below are the recommended post-care instructions:

1. **Hygiene**
   Always wash your hands before touching your eyebrows.
   For the first week, gently cleanse the treated area with lukewarm water.
   Soak a cotton pad in lukewarm water and gently dab your eyebrows, avoiding any rubbing motions.
   Dry the area using a dry cotton pad, again with gentle dabbing to avoid friction.
   Repeat this process 4 times a day at regular intervals.
   For the first two weeks, avoid excessive moisture on the eyebrows (e.g., during baths or showers). After 7-14 days, when the initial healing has occurred, you may begin using a gentle micellar water for cleansing. Avoid products containing alcohol or harsh ingredients.

2. **Preventing Irritation**
   Do not scratch or rub your eyebrows, even if small scabs form. Allow the scabs to fall off naturally to avoid scarring or pigment loss.
   Avoid applying makeup to the eyebrow area until fully healed (approximately 7-14 days).
   For at least 14 days, avoid saunas, swimming pools, hot baths, and excessive sweating, as these can cause the pigment to fade or irritate the skin.

3. **Sun Protection**
   Avoid sun exposure and tanning beds for at least 4 weeks. UV radiation can cause the pigment to fade.
   Once your eyebrows are fully healed, apply a high SPF sunscreen to protect the pigment from fading.

4. **Avoiding Intensive Cosmetic Treatments**
   For 4-6 weeks post-procedure, avoid facial treatments such as chemical peels, laser treatments, or the use of strong creams around the eyebrow area, as these may weaken the pigment.

5. **Consulting a Specialist**
   If you have any concerns or notice unusual symptoms such as excessive redness, swelling, or oozing, contact the cosmetologist who performed the procedure.

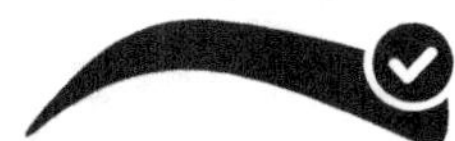

Healing process after micropigmentation

The healing process following permanent eyebrow makeup takes place in several stages and usually lasts between 4 to 6 weeks. During this time, the appearance of your eyebrows will change as the pigment gradually settles into the skin. Below are the stages of the healing process:

1. **Day 1: Immediately After the Procedure**

   Your eyebrows will look very intense, dark, and prominent. The skin may be slightly swollen and red. The pigment will appear darker than the final result, as the dye is still on the surface of the skin.

2. **Days 2–3**

   Swelling starts to subside, and the skin around the eyebrows may feel dry or tight.
   The eyebrows will still appear dark, but the skin begins to form a light protective layer.

3. **Days 4–7**

   Exfoliation begins. Scabs may form and fall off naturally, so it's important not to touch, scratch, or try to speed up the process.
   Your eyebrows may look uneven or have „empty" spots, but this is a normal part of healing as the pigment settles.

4. **Days 7–14**

   The scabs gradually fall off, and the pigment may look much lighter. Many people feel that their eyebrows are too light at this stage, but the color will continue to stabilize.
   Continue to avoid excessive washing and using cosmetics on the eyebrow area.

5. **Days 14–21**

   The eyebrows will appear lighter and more natural. Some areas may seem lighter than others, but this is part of the process.
   The pigment begins to settle into the skin, and the final color will start to become more visible.

6. **After 4 Weeks**

   By this point, the eyebrows are fully healed. The color will be 20-50% lighter compared to the first few days post-procedure.
   A touch-up session may be needed to fill any pigment gaps or refine the shape.

Date of your touch-up:

Post-procedure care after micropigmentation

Following a micropigmentation procedure, the skin requires special attention to ensure proper healing and long-lasting, aesthetic results. Below are the recommended post-care instructions:

1. **Hygiene**

   Always wash your hands before touching your eyebrows.

   For the first week, gently cleanse the treated area with lukewarm water.

   Soak a cotton pad in lukewarm water and gently dab your eyebrows, avoiding any rubbing motions.

   Dry the area using a dry cotton pad, again with gentle dabbing to avoid friction.

   Repeat this process 4 times a day at regular intervals.

   For the first two weeks, avoid excessive moisture on the eyebrows (e.g., during baths or showers). After 7-14 days, when the initial healing has occurred, you may begin using a gentle micellar water for cleansing. Avoid products containing alcohol or harsh ingredients.

2. **Preventing Irritation**

   Do not scratch or rub your eyebrows, even if small scabs form. Allow the scabs to fall off naturally to avoid scarring or pigment loss.

   Avoid applying makeup to the eyebrow area until fully healed (approximately 7-14 days).

   For at least 14 days, avoid saunas, swimming pools, hot baths, and excessive sweating, as these can cause the pigment to fade or irritate the skin.

3. **Sun Protection**

   Avoid sun exposure and tanning beds for at least 4 weeks. UV radiation can cause the pigment to fade.

   Once your eyebrows are fully healed, apply a high SPF sunscreen to protect the pigment from fading.

4. **Avoiding Intensive Cosmetic Treatments**

   For 4-6 weeks post-procedure, avoid facial treatments such as chemical peels, laser treatments, or the use of strong creams around the eyebrow area, as these may weaken the pigment.

5. **Consulting a Specialist**

   If you have any concerns or notice unusual symptoms such as excessive redness, swelling, or oozing, contact the cosmetologist who performed the procedure.

Healing process after micropigmentation

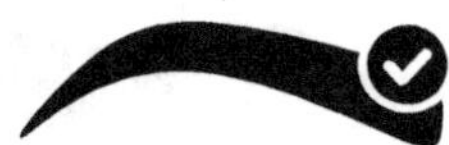

The healing process following permanent eyebrow makeup takes place in several stages and usually lasts between 4 to 6 weeks. During this time, the appearance of your eyebrows will change as the pigment gradually settles into the skin. Below are the stages of the healing process:

1. **Day 1: Immediately After the Procedure**
   Your eyebrows will look very intense, dark, and prominent. The skin may be slightly swollen and red. The pigment will appear darker than the final result, as the dye is still on the surface of the skin.

2. **Days 2–3**
   Swelling starts to subside, and the skin around the eyebrows may feel dry or tight.
   The eyebrows will still appear dark, but the skin begins to form a light protective layer.

3. **Days 4–7**
   Exfoliation begins. Scabs may form and fall off naturally, so it's important not to touch, scratch, or try to speed up the process.
   Your eyebrows may look uneven or have „empty" spots, but this is a normal part of healing as the pigment settles.

4. **Days 7–14**
   The scabs gradually fall off, and the pigment may look much lighter. Many people feel that their eyebrows are too light at this stage, but the color will continue to stabilize.
   Continue to avoid excessive washing and using cosmetics on the eyebrow area.

5. **Days 14–21**
   The eyebrows will appear lighter and more natural. Some areas may seem lighter than others, but this is part of the process.
   The pigment begins to settle into the skin, and the final color will start to become more visible.

6. **After 4 Weeks**
   By this point, the eyebrows are fully healed. The color will be 20-50% lighter compared to the first few days post-procedure.
   A touch-up session may be needed to fill any pigment gaps or refine the shape.

Date of your touch-up:

Post-procedure care after micropigmentation

Following a micropigmentation procedure, the skin requires special attention to ensure proper healing and long-lasting, aesthetic results. Below are the recommended post-care instructions:

1. **Hygiene**
   Always wash your hands before touching your eyebrows.
   For the first week, gently cleanse the treated area with lukewarm water.
   Soak a cotton pad in lukewarm water and gently dab your eyebrows, avoiding any rubbing motions.
   Dry the area using a dry cotton pad, again with gentle dabbing to avoid friction.
   Repeat this process 4 times a day at regular intervals.
   For the first two weeks, avoid excessive moisture on the eyebrows (e.g., during baths or showers). After 7-14 days, when the initial healing has occurred, you may begin using a gentle micellar water for cleansing. Avoid products containing alcohol or harsh ingredients.

2. **Preventing Irritation**
   Do not scratch or rub your eyebrows, even if small scabs form. Allow the scabs to fall off naturally to avoid scarring or pigment loss.
   Avoid applying makeup to the eyebrow area until fully healed (approximately 7-14 days).
   For at least 14 days, avoid saunas, swimming pools, hot baths, and excessive sweating, as these can cause the pigment to fade or irritate the skin.

3. **Sun Protection**
   Avoid sun exposure and tanning beds for at least 4 weeks. UV radiation can cause the pigment to fade.
   Once your eyebrows are fully healed, apply a high SPF sunscreen to protect the pigment from fading.

4. **Avoiding Intensive Cosmetic Treatments**
   For 4-6 weeks post-procedure, avoid facial treatments such as chemical peels, laser treatments, or the use of strong creams around the eyebrow area, as these may weaken the pigment.

5. **Consulting a Specialist**
   If you have any concerns or notice unusual symptoms such as excessive redness, swelling, or oozing, contact the cosmetologist who performed the procedure.

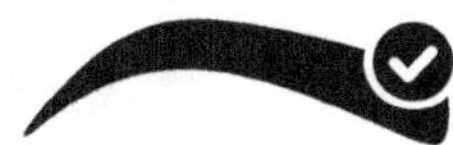

Healing process after micropigmentation

The healing process following permanent eyebrow makeup takes place in several stages and usually lasts between 4 to 6 weeks. During this time, the appearance of your eyebrows will change as the pigment gradually settles into the skin. Below are the stages of the healing process:

1. **Day 1: Immediately After the Procedure**
   Your eyebrows will look very intense, dark, and prominent. The skin may be slightly swollen and red. The pigment will appear darker than the final result, as the dye is still on the surface of the skin.

2. **Days 2–3**
   Swelling starts to subside, and the skin around the eyebrows may feel dry or tight.
   The eyebrows will still appear dark, but the skin begins to form a light protective layer.

3. **Days 4–7**
   Exfoliation begins. Scabs may form and fall off naturally, so it's important not to touch, scratch, or try to speed up the process.
   Your eyebrows may look uneven or have „empty" spots, but this is a normal part of healing as the pigment settles.

4. **Days 7–14**
   The scabs gradually fall off, and the pigment may look much lighter. Many people feel that their eyebrows are too light at this stage, but the color will continue to stabilize.
   Continue to avoid excessive washing and using cosmetics on the eyebrow area.

5. **Days 14–21**
   The eyebrows will appear lighter and more natural. Some areas may seem lighter than others, but this is part of the process.
   The pigment begins to settle into the skin, and the final color will start to become more visible.

6. **After 4 Weeks**
   By this point, the eyebrows are fully healed. The color will be 20-50% lighter compared to the first few days post-procedure.
   A touch-up session may be needed to fill any pigment gaps or refine the shape.

Date of your touch-up:

Post-procedure care after micropigmentation

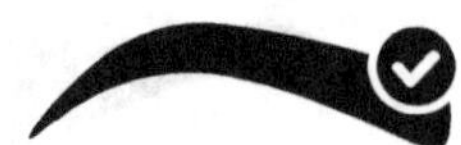

Following a micropigmentation procedure, the skin requires special attention to ensure proper healing and long-lasting, aesthetic results. Below are the recommended post-care instructions:

1. **Hygiene**
   Always wash your hands before touching your eyebrows.
   For the first week, gently cleanse the treated area with lukewarm water.
   Soak a cotton pad in lukewarm water and gently dab your eyebrows, avoiding any rubbing motions.
   Dry the area using a dry cotton pad, again with gentle dabbing to avoid friction.
   Repeat this process 4 times a day at regular intervals.
   For the first two weeks, avoid excessive moisture on the eyebrows (e.g., during baths or showers). After 7-14 days, when the initial healing has occurred, you may begin using a gentle micellar water for cleansing. Avoid products containing alcohol or harsh ingredients.

2. **Preventing Irritation**
   Do not scratch or rub your eyebrows, even if small scabs form. Allow the scabs to fall off naturally to avoid scarring or pigment loss.
   Avoid applying makeup to the eyebrow area until fully healed (approximately 7-14 days).
   For at least 14 days, avoid saunas, swimming pools, hot baths, and excessive sweating, as these can cause the pigment to fade or irritate the skin.

3. **Sun Protection**
   Avoid sun exposure and tanning beds for at least 4 weeks. UV radiation can cause the pigment to fade.
   Once your eyebrows are fully healed, apply a high SPF sunscreen to protect the pigment from fading.

4. **Avoiding Intensive Cosmetic Treatments**
   For 4-6 weeks post-procedure, avoid facial treatments such as chemical peels, laser treatments, or the use of strong creams around the eyebrow area, as these may weaken the pigment.

5. **Consulting a Specialist**
   If you have any concerns or notice unusual symptoms such as excessive redness, swelling, or oozing, contact the cosmetologist who performed the procedure.

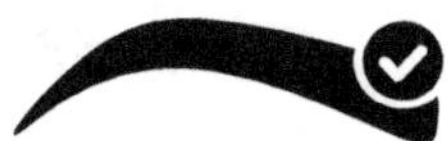

Healing process after micropigmentation

The healing process following permanent eyebrow makeup takes place in several stages and usually lasts between 4 to 6 weeks. During this time, the appearance of your eyebrows will change as the pigment gradually settles into the skin. Below are the stages of the healing process:

1. **Day 1: Immediately After the Procedure**
   Your eyebrows will look very intense, dark, and prominent. The skin may be slightly swollen and red. The pigment will appear darker than the final result, as the dye is still on the surface of the skin.

2. **Days 2–3**
   Swelling starts to subside, and the skin around the eyebrows may feel dry or tight.
   The eyebrows will still appear dark, but the skin begins to form a light protective layer.

3. **Days 4–7**
   Exfoliation begins. Scabs may form and fall off naturally, so it's important not to touch, scratch, or try to speed up the process.
   Your eyebrows may look uneven or have „empty" spots, but this is a normal part of healing as the pigment settles.

4. **Days 7–14**
   The scabs gradually fall off, and the pigment may look much lighter. Many people feel that their eyebrows are too light at this stage, but the color will continue to stabilize.
   Continue to avoid excessive washing and using cosmetics on the eyebrow area.

5. **Days 14–21**
   The eyebrows will appear lighter and more natural. Some areas may seem lighter than others, but this is part of the process.
   The pigment begins to settle into the skin, and the final color will start to become more visible.

6. **After 4 Weeks**
   By this point, the eyebrows are fully healed. The color will be 20-50% lighter compared to the first few days post-procedure.
   A touch-up session may be needed to fill any pigment gaps or refine the shape.

Date of your touch-up:

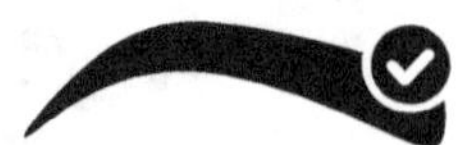

Post-procedure care after micropigmentation

Following a micropigmentation procedure, the skin requires special attention to ensure proper healing and long-lasting, aesthetic results. Below are the recommended post-care instructions:

1. **Hygiene**

   Always wash your hands before touching your eyebrows.

   For the first week, gently cleanse the treated area with lukewarm water.

   Soak a cotton pad in lukewarm water and gently dab your eyebrows, avoiding any rubbing motions.

   Dry the area using a dry cotton pad, again with gentle dabbing to avoid friction.

   Repeat this process 4 times a day at regular intervals.

   For the first two weeks, avoid excessive moisture on the eyebrows (e.g., during baths or showers). After 7-14 days, when the initial healing has occurred, you may begin using a gentle micellar water for cleansing. Avoid products containing alcohol or harsh ingredients.

2. **Preventing Irritation**

   Do not scratch or rub your eyebrows, even if small scabs form. Allow the scabs to fall off naturally to avoid scarring or pigment loss.

   Avoid applying makeup to the eyebrow area until fully healed (approximately 7-14 days).

   For at least 14 days, avoid saunas, swimming pools, hot baths, and excessive sweating, as these can cause the pigment to fade or irritate the skin.

3. **Sun Protection**

   Avoid sun exposure and tanning beds for at least 4 weeks. UV radiation can cause the pigment to fade.

   Once your eyebrows are fully healed, apply a high SPF sunscreen to protect the pigment from fading.

4. **Avoiding Intensive Cosmetic Treatments**

   For 4-6 weeks post-procedure, avoid facial treatments such as chemical peels, laser treatments, or the use of strong creams around the eyebrow area, as these may weaken the pigment.

5. **Consulting a Specialist**

   If you have any concerns or notice unusual symptoms such as excessive redness, swelling, or oozing, contact the cosmetologist who performed the procedure.

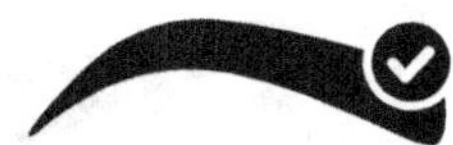

Healing process after micropigmentation

The healing process following permanent eyebrow makeup takes place in several stages and usually lasts between 4 to 6 weeks. During this time, the appearance of your eyebrows will change as the pigment gradually settles into the skin. Below are the stages of the healing process:

1. **Day 1: Immediately After the Procedure**
   Your eyebrows will look very intense, dark, and prominent. The skin may be slightly swollen and red. The pigment will appear darker than the final result, as the dye is still on the surface of the skin.

2. **Days 2–3**
   Swelling starts to subside, and the skin around the eyebrows may feel dry or tight.
   The eyebrows will still appear dark, but the skin begins to form a light protective layer.

3. **Days 4–7**
   Exfoliation begins. Scabs may form and fall off naturally, so it's important not to touch, scratch, or try to speed up the process.
   Your eyebrows may look uneven or have „empty" spots, but this is a normal part of healing as the pigment settles.

4. **Days 7–14**
   The scabs gradually fall off, and the pigment may look much lighter. Many people feel that their eyebrows are too light at this stage, but the color will continue to stabilize.
   Continue to avoid excessive washing and using cosmetics on the eyebrow area.

5. **Days 14–21**
   The eyebrows will appear lighter and more natural. Some areas may seem lighter than others, but this is part of the process.
   The pigment begins to settle into the skin, and the final color will start to become more visible.

6. **After 4 Weeks**
   By this point, the eyebrows are fully healed. The color will be 20-50% lighter compared to the first few days post-procedure.
   A touch-up session may be needed to fill any pigment gaps or refine the shape.

Date of your touch-up:

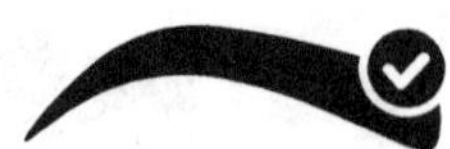

Post-procedure care after micropigmentation

Following a micropigmentation procedure, the skin requires special attention to ensure proper healing and long-lasting, aesthetic results. Below are the recommended post-care instructions:

1. **Hygiene**

   Always wash your hands before touching your eyebrows.

   For the first week, gently cleanse the treated area with lukewarm water.

   Soak a cotton pad in lukewarm water and gently dab your eyebrows, avoiding any rubbing motions.

   Dry the area using a dry cotton pad, again with gentle dabbing to avoid friction.

   Repeat this process 4 times a day at regular intervals.

   For the first two weeks, avoid excessive moisture on the eyebrows (e.g., during baths or showers). After 7-14 days, when the initial healing has occurred, you may begin using a gentle micellar water for cleansing. Avoid products containing alcohol or harsh ingredients.

2. **Preventing Irritation**

   Do not scratch or rub your eyebrows, even if small scabs form. Allow the scabs to fall off naturally to avoid scarring or pigment loss.

   Avoid applying makeup to the eyebrow area until fully healed (approximately 7-14 days).

   For at least 14 days, avoid saunas, swimming pools, hot baths, and excessive sweating, as these can cause the pigment to fade or irritate the skin.

3. **Sun Protection**

   Avoid sun exposure and tanning beds for at least 4 weeks. UV radiation can cause the pigment to fade.

   Once your eyebrows are fully healed, apply a high SPF sunscreen to protect the pigment from fading.

4. **Avoiding Intensive Cosmetic Treatments**

   For 4-6 weeks post-procedure, avoid facial treatments such as chemical peels, laser treatments, or the use of strong creams around the eyebrow area, as these may weaken the pigment.

5. **Consulting a Specialist**

   If you have any concerns or notice unusual symptoms such as excessive redness, swelling, or oozing, contact the cosmetologist who performed the procedure.

Healing process after micropigmentation

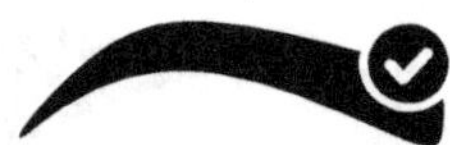

The healing process following permanent eyebrow makeup takes place in several stages and usually lasts between 4 to 6 weeks. During this time, the appearance of your eyebrows will change as the pigment gradually settles into the skin. Below are the stages of the healing process:

1. **Day 1: Immediately After the Procedure**
   Your eyebrows will look very intense, dark, and prominent. The skin may be slightly swollen and red. The pigment will appear darker than the final result, as the dye is still on the surface of the skin.

2. **Days 2–3**
   Swelling starts to subside, and the skin around the eyebrows may feel dry or tight.
   The eyebrows will still appear dark, but the skin begins to form a light protective layer.

3. **Days 4–7**
   Exfoliation begins. Scabs may form and fall off naturally, so it's important not to touch, scratch, or try to speed up the process.
   Your eyebrows may look uneven or have „empty" spots, but this is a normal part of healing as the pigment settles.

4. **Days 7–14**
   The scabs gradually fall off, and the pigment may look much lighter. Many people feel that their eyebrows are too light at this stage, but the color will continue to stabilize.
   Continue to avoid excessive washing and using cosmetics on the eyebrow area.

5. **Days 14–21**
   The eyebrows will appear lighter and more natural. Some areas may seem lighter than others, but this is part of the process.
   The pigment begins to settle into the skin, and the final color will start to become more visible.

6. **After 4 Weeks**
   By this point, the eyebrows are fully healed. The color will be 20-50% lighter compared to the first few days post-procedure.
   A touch-up session may be needed to fill any pigment gaps or refine the shape.

Date of your touch-up:

Post-procedure care after micropigmentation

Following a micropigmentation procedure, the skin requires special attention to ensure proper healing and long-lasting, aesthetic results. Below are the recommended post-care instructions:

1. **Hygiene**
   Always wash your hands before touching your eyebrows.
   For the first week, gently cleanse the treated area with lukewarm water.
   Soak a cotton pad in lukewarm water and gently dab your eyebrows, avoiding any rubbing motions.
   Dry the area using a dry cotton pad, again with gentle dabbing to avoid friction.
   Repeat this process 4 times a day at regular intervals.
   For the first two weeks, avoid excessive moisture on the eyebrows (e.g., during baths or showers). After 7-14 days, when the initial healing has occurred, you may begin using a gentle micellar water for cleansing. Avoid products containing alcohol or harsh ingredients.

2. **Preventing Irritation**
   Do not scratch or rub your eyebrows, even if small scabs form. Allow the scabs to fall off naturally to avoid scarring or pigment loss.
   Avoid applying makeup to the eyebrow area until fully healed (approximately 7-14 days).
   For at least 14 days, avoid saunas, swimming pools, hot baths, and excessive sweating, as these can cause the pigment to fade or irritate the skin.

3. **Sun Protection**
   Avoid sun exposure and tanning beds for at least 4 weeks. UV radiation can cause the pigment to fade.
   Once your eyebrows are fully healed, apply a high SPF sunscreen to protect the pigment from fading.

4. **Avoiding Intensive Cosmetic Treatments**
   For 4-6 weeks post-procedure, avoid facial treatments such as chemical peels, laser treatments, or the use of strong creams around the eyebrow area, as these may weaken the pigment.

5. **Consulting a Specialist**
   If you have any concerns or notice unusual symptoms such as excessive redness, swelling, or oozing, contact the cosmetologist who performed the procedure.

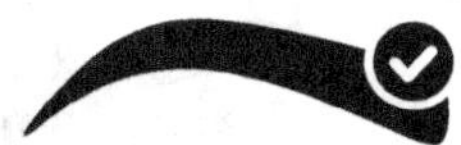

Healing process after micropigmentation

The healing process following permanent eyebrow makeup takes place in several stages and usually lasts between 4 to 6 weeks. During this time, the appearance of your eyebrows will change as the pigment gradually settles into the skin. Below are the stages of the healing process:

1. **Day 1: Immediately After the Procedure**
   Your eyebrows will look very intense, dark, and prominent. The skin may be slightly swollen and red. The pigment will appear darker than the final result, as the dye is still on the surface of the skin.

2. **Days 2–3**
   Swelling starts to subside, and the skin around the eyebrows may feel dry or tight.
   The eyebrows will still appear dark, but the skin begins to form a light protective layer.

3. **Days 4–7**
   Exfoliation begins. Scabs may form and fall off naturally, so it's important not to touch, scratch, or try to speed up the process.
   Your eyebrows may look uneven or have „empty" spots, but this is a normal part of healing as the pigment settles.

4. **Days 7–14**
   The scabs gradually fall off, and the pigment may look much lighter. Many people feel that their eyebrows are too light at this stage, but the color will continue to stabilize.
   Continue to avoid excessive washing and using cosmetics on the eyebrow area.

5. **Days 14–21**
   The eyebrows will appear lighter and more natural. Some areas may seem lighter than others, but this is part of the process.
   The pigment begins to settle into the skin, and the final color will start to become more visible.

6. **After 4 Weeks**
   By this point, the eyebrows are fully healed. The color will be 20-50% lighter compared to the first few days post-procedure.
   A touch-up session may be needed to fill any pigment gaps or refine the shape.

Date of your touch-up:

Post-procedure care after micropigmentation

Following a micropigmentation procedure, the skin requires special attention to ensure proper healing and long-lasting, aesthetic results. Below are the recommended post-care instructions:

1. **Hygiene**
   Always wash your hands before touching your eyebrows.
   For the first week, gently cleanse the treated area with lukewarm water.
   Soak a cotton pad in lukewarm water and gently dab your eyebrows, avoiding any rubbing motions.
   Dry the area using a dry cotton pad, again with gentle dabbing to avoid friction.
   Repeat this process 4 times a day at regular intervals.
   For the first two weeks, avoid excessive moisture on the eyebrows (e.g., during baths or showers). After 7-14 days, when the initial healing has occurred, you may begin using a gentle micellar water for cleansing. Avoid products containing alcohol or harsh ingredients.

2. **Preventing Irritation**
   Do not scratch or rub your eyebrows, even if small scabs form. Allow the scabs to fall off naturally to avoid scarring or pigment loss.
   Avoid applying makeup to the eyebrow area until fully healed (approximately 7-14 days).
   For at least 14 days, avoid saunas, swimming pools, hot baths, and excessive sweating, as these can cause the pigment to fade or irritate the skin.

3. **Sun Protection**
   Avoid sun exposure and tanning beds for at least 4 weeks. UV radiation can cause the pigment to fade.
   Once your eyebrows are fully healed, apply a high SPF sunscreen to protect the pigment from fading.

4. **Avoiding Intensive Cosmetic Treatments**
   For 4-6 weeks post-procedure, avoid facial treatments such as chemical peels, laser treatments, or the use of strong creams around the eyebrow area, as these may weaken the pigment.

5. **Consulting a Specialist**
   If you have any concerns or notice unusual symptoms such as excessive redness, swelling, or oozing, contact the cosmetologist who performed the procedure.

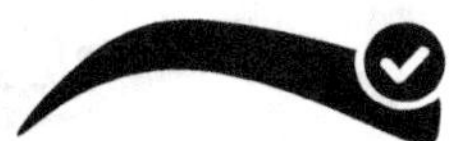

Healing process after micropigmentation

The healing process following permanent eyebrow makeup takes place in several stages and usually lasts between 4 to 6 weeks. During this time, the appearance of your eyebrows will change as the pigment gradually settles into the skin. Below are the stages of the healing process:

1. **Day 1: Immediately After the Procedure**
   Your eyebrows will look very intense, dark, and prominent. The skin may be slightly swollen and red. The pigment will appear darker than the final result, as the dye is still on the surface of the skin.

2. **Days 2–3**
   Swelling starts to subside, and the skin around the eyebrows may feel dry or tight.
   The eyebrows will still appear dark, but the skin begins to form a light protective layer.

3. **Days 4–7**
   Exfoliation begins. Scabs may form and fall off naturally, so it's important not to touch, scratch, or try to speed up the process.
   Your eyebrows may look uneven or have „empty" spots, but this is a normal part of healing as the pigment settles.

4. **Days 7–14**
   The scabs gradually fall off, and the pigment may look much lighter. Many people feel that their eyebrows are too light at this stage, but the color will continue to stabilize.
   Continue to avoid excessive washing and using cosmetics on the eyebrow area.

5. **Days 14–21**
   The eyebrows will appear lighter and more natural. Some areas may seem lighter than others, but this is part of the process.
   The pigment begins to settle into the skin, and the final color will start to become more visible.

6. **After 4 Weeks**
   By this point, the eyebrows are fully healed. The color will be 20-50% lighter compared to the first few days post-procedure.
   A touch-up session may be needed to fill any pigment gaps or refine the shape.

Date of your touch-up:

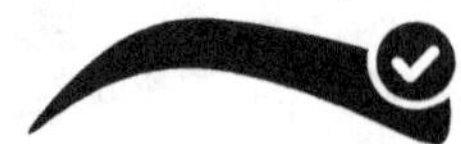

Post-procedure care after micropigmentation

Following a micropigmentation procedure, the skin requires special attention to ensure proper healing and long-lasting, aesthetic results. Below are the recommended post-care instructions:

1. **Hygiene**

   Always wash your hands before touching your eyebrows.

   For the first week, gently cleanse the treated area with lukewarm water.

   Soak a cotton pad in lukewarm water and gently dab your eyebrows, avoiding any rubbing motions.

   Dry the area using a dry cotton pad, again with gentle dabbing to avoid friction.

   Repeat this process 4 times a day at regular intervals.

   For the first two weeks, avoid excessive moisture on the eyebrows (e.g., during baths or showers). After 7-14 days, when the initial healing has occurred, you may begin using a gentle micellar water for cleansing. Avoid products containing alcohol or harsh ingredients.

2. **Preventing Irritation**

   Do not scratch or rub your eyebrows, even if small scabs form. Allow the scabs to fall off naturally to avoid scarring or pigment loss.

   Avoid applying makeup to the eyebrow area until fully healed (approximately 7-14 days).

   For at least 14 days, avoid saunas, swimming pools, hot baths, and excessive sweating, as these can cause the pigment to fade or irritate the skin.

3. **Sun Protection**

   Avoid sun exposure and tanning beds for at least 4 weeks. UV radiation can cause the pigment to fade.

   Once your eyebrows are fully healed, apply a high SPF sunscreen to protect the pigment from fading.

4. **Avoiding Intensive Cosmetic Treatments**

   For 4-6 weeks post-procedure, avoid facial treatments such as chemical peels, laser treatments, or the use of strong creams around the eyebrow area, as these may weaken the pigment.

5. **Consulting a Specialist**

   If you have any concerns or notice unusual symptoms such as excessive redness, swelling, or oozing, contact the cosmetologist who performed the procedure.

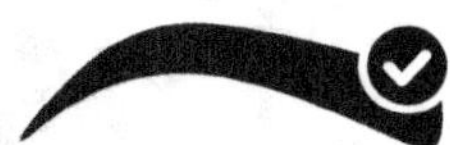

Healing process after micropigmentation

The healing process following permanent eyebrow makeup takes place in several stages and usually lasts between 4 to 6 weeks. During this time, the appearance of your eyebrows will change as the pigment gradually settles into the skin. Below are the stages of the healing process:

1. **Day 1: Immediately After the Procedure**
   Your eyebrows will look very intense, dark, and prominent. The skin may be slightly swollen and red. The pigment will appear darker than the final result, as the dye is still on the surface of the skin.

2. **Days 2–3**
   Swelling starts to subside, and the skin around the eyebrows may feel dry or tight.
   The eyebrows will still appear dark, but the skin begins to form a light protective layer.

3. **Days 4–7**
   Exfoliation begins. Scabs may form and fall off naturally, so it's important not to touch, scratch, or try to speed up the process.
   Your eyebrows may look uneven or have „empty" spots, but this is a normal part of healing as the pigment settles.

4. **Days 7–14**
   The scabs gradually fall off, and the pigment may look much lighter. Many people feel that their eyebrows are too light at this stage, but the color will continue to stabilize.
   Continue to avoid excessive washing and using cosmetics on the eyebrow area.

5. **Days 14–21**
   The eyebrows will appear lighter and more natural. Some areas may seem lighter than others, but this is part of the process.
   The pigment begins to settle into the skin, and the final color will start to become more visible.

6. **After 4 Weeks**
   By this point, the eyebrows are fully healed. The color will be 20-50% lighter compared to the first few days post-procedure.
   A touch-up session may be needed to fill any pigment gaps or refine the shape.

Date of your touch-up:

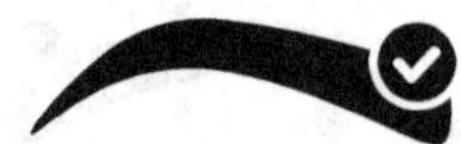

Post-procedure care after micropigmentation

Following a micropigmentation procedure, the skin requires special attention to ensure proper healing and long-lasting, aesthetic results. Below are the recommended post-care instructions:

1. **Hygiene**

   Always wash your hands before touching your eyebrows.

   For the first week, gently cleanse the treated area with lukewarm water.

   Soak a cotton pad in lukewarm water and gently dab your eyebrows, avoiding any rubbing motions.

   Dry the area using a dry cotton pad, again with gentle dabbing to avoid friction.

   Repeat this process 4 times a day at regular intervals.

   For the first two weeks, avoid excessive moisture on the eyebrows (e.g., during baths or showers). After 7-14 days, when the initial healing has occurred, you may begin using a gentle micellar water for cleansing. Avoid products containing alcohol or harsh ingredients.

2. **Preventing Irritation**

   Do not scratch or rub your eyebrows, even if small scabs form. Allow the scabs to fall off naturally to avoid scarring or pigment loss.

   Avoid applying makeup to the eyebrow area until fully healed (approximately 7-14 days).

   For at least 14 days, avoid saunas, swimming pools, hot baths, and excessive sweating, as these can cause the pigment to fade or irritate the skin.

3. **Sun Protection**

   Avoid sun exposure and tanning beds for at least 4 weeks. UV radiation can cause the pigment to fade.

   Once your eyebrows are fully healed, apply a high SPF sunscreen to protect the pigment from fading.

4. **Avoiding Intensive Cosmetic Treatments**

   For 4-6 weeks post-procedure, avoid facial treatments such as chemical peels, laser treatments, or the use of strong creams around the eyebrow area, as these may weaken the pigment.

5. **Consulting a Specialist**

   If you have any concerns or notice unusual symptoms such as excessive redness, swelling, or oozing, contact the cosmetologist who performed the procedure.

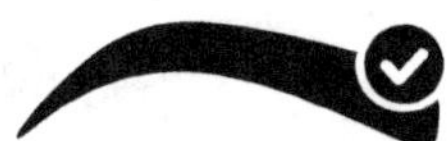

Healing process after micropigmentation

The healing process following permanent eyebrow makeup takes place in several stages and usually lasts between 4 to 6 weeks. During this time, the appearance of your eyebrows will change as the pigment gradually settles into the skin. Below are the stages of the healing process:

1. **Day 1: Immediately After the Procedure**
   Your eyebrows will look very intense, dark, and prominent. The skin may be slightly swollen and red. The pigment will appear darker than the final result, as the dye is still on the surface of the skin.

2. **Days 2–3**
   Swelling starts to subside, and the skin around the eyebrows may feel dry or tight.
   The eyebrows will still appear dark, but the skin begins to form a light protective layer.

3. **Days 4–7**
   Exfoliation begins. Scabs may form and fall off naturally, so it's important not to touch, scratch, or try to speed up the process.
   Your eyebrows may look uneven or have „empty" spots, but this is a normal part of healing as the pigment settles.

4. **Days 7–14**
   The scabs gradually fall off, and the pigment may look much lighter. Many people feel that their eyebrows are too light at this stage, but the color will continue to stabilize.
   Continue to avoid excessive washing and using cosmetics on the eyebrow area.

5. **Days 14–21**
   The eyebrows will appear lighter and more natural. Some areas may seem lighter than others, but this is part of the process.
   The pigment begins to settle into the skin, and the final color will start to become more visible.

6. **After 4 Weeks**
   By this point, the eyebrows are fully healed. The color will be 20-50% lighter compared to the first few days post-procedure.
   A touch-up session may be needed to fill any pigment gaps or refine the shape.

Date of your touch-up:

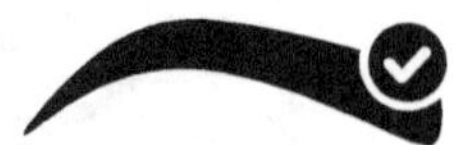

Post-procedure care after micropigmentation

Following a micropigmentation procedure, the skin requires special attention to ensure proper healing and long-lasting, aesthetic results. Below are the recommended post-care instructions:

1. **Hygiene**

   Always wash your hands before touching your eyebrows.

   For the first week, gently cleanse the treated area with lukewarm water.

   Soak a cotton pad in lukewarm water and gently dab your eyebrows, avoiding any rubbing motions.

   Dry the area using a dry cotton pad, again with gentle dabbing to avoid friction.

   Repeat this process 4 times a day at regular intervals.

   For the first two weeks, avoid excessive moisture on the eyebrows (e.g., during baths or showers). After 7-14 days, when the initial healing has occurred, you may begin using a gentle micellar water for cleansing. Avoid products containing alcohol or harsh ingredients.

2. **Preventing Irritation**

   Do not scratch or rub your eyebrows, even if small scabs form. Allow the scabs to fall off naturally to avoid scarring or pigment loss.

   Avoid applying makeup to the eyebrow area until fully healed (approximately 7-14 days).

   For at least 14 days, avoid saunas, swimming pools, hot baths, and excessive sweating, as these can cause the pigment to fade or irritate the skin.

3. **Sun Protection**

   Avoid sun exposure and tanning beds for at least 4 weeks. UV radiation can cause the pigment to fade.

   Once your eyebrows are fully healed, apply a high SPF sunscreen to protect the pigment from fading.

4. **Avoiding Intensive Cosmetic Treatments**

   For 4-6 weeks post-procedure, avoid facial treatments such as chemical peels, laser treatments, or the use of strong creams around the eyebrow area, as these may weaken the pigment.

5. **Consulting a Specialist**

   If you have any concerns or notice unusual symptoms such as excessive redness, swelling, or oozing, contact the cosmetologist who performed the procedure.

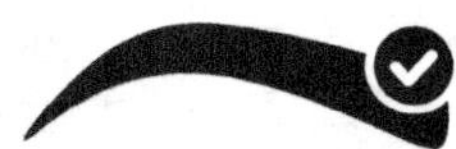

Healing process after micropigmentation

The healing process following permanent eyebrow makeup takes place in several stages and usually lasts between 4 to 6 weeks. During this time, the appearance of your eyebrows will change as the pigment gradually settles into the skin. Below are the stages of the healing process:

1. **Day 1: Immediately After the Procedure**
   Your eyebrows will look very intense, dark, and prominent. The skin may be slightly swollen and red. The pigment will appear darker than the final result, as the dye is still on the surface of the skin.

2. **Days 2–3**
   Swelling starts to subside, and the skin around the eyebrows may feel dry or tight.
   The eyebrows will still appear dark, but the skin begins to form a light protective layer.

3. **Days 4–7**
   Exfoliation begins. Scabs may form and fall off naturally, so it's important not to touch, scratch, or try to speed up the process.
   Your eyebrows may look uneven or have „empty" spots, but this is a normal part of healing as the pigment settles.

4. **Days 7–14**
   The scabs gradually fall off, and the pigment may look much lighter. Many people feel that their eyebrows are too light at this stage, but the color will continue to stabilize.
   Continue to avoid excessive washing and using cosmetics on the eyebrow area.

5. **Days 14–21**
   The eyebrows will appear lighter and more natural. Some areas may seem lighter than others, but this is part of the process.
   The pigment begins to settle into the skin, and the final color will start to become more visible.

6. **After 4 Weeks**
   By this point, the eyebrows are fully healed. The color will be 20-50% lighter compared to the first few days post-procedure.
   A touch-up session may be needed to fill any pigment gaps or refine the shape.

Date of your touch-up:

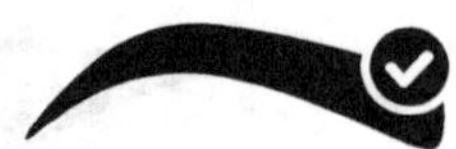

Post-procedure care after micropigmentation

Following a micropigmentation procedure, the skin requires special attention to ensure proper healing and long-lasting, aesthetic results. Below are the recommended post-care instructions:

1. **Hygiene**
   Always wash your hands before touching your eyebrows.
   For the first week, gently cleanse the treated area with lukewarm water.
   Soak a cotton pad in lukewarm water and gently dab your eyebrows, avoiding any rubbing motions.
   Dry the area using a dry cotton pad, again with gentle dabbing to avoid friction.
   Repeat this process 4 times a day at regular intervals.
   For the first two weeks, avoid excessive moisture on the eyebrows (e.g., during baths or showers). After 7-14 days, when the initial healing has occurred, you may begin using a gentle micellar water for cleansing. Avoid products containing alcohol or harsh ingredients.

2. **Preventing Irritation**
   Do not scratch or rub your eyebrows, even if small scabs form. Allow the scabs to fall off naturally to avoid scarring or pigment loss.
   Avoid applying makeup to the eyebrow area until fully healed (approximately 7-14 days).
   For at least 14 days, avoid saunas, swimming pools, hot baths, and excessive sweating, as these can cause the pigment to fade or irritate the skin.

3. **Sun Protection**
   Avoid sun exposure and tanning beds for at least 4 weeks. UV radiation can cause the pigment to fade.
   Once your eyebrows are fully healed, apply a high SPF sunscreen to protect the pigment from fading.

4. **Avoiding Intensive Cosmetic Treatments**
   For 4-6 weeks post-procedure, avoid facial treatments such as chemical peels, laser treatments, or the use of strong creams around the eyebrow area, as these may weaken the pigment.

5. **Consulting a Specialist**
   If you have any concerns or notice unusual symptoms such as excessive redness, swelling, or oozing, contact the cosmetologist who performed the procedure.

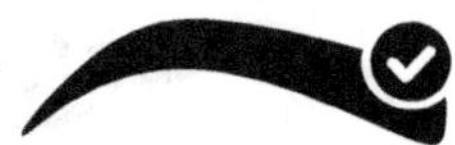

Healing process after micropigmentation

The healing process following permanent eyebrow makeup takes place in several stages and usually lasts between 4 to 6 weeks. During this time, the appearance of your eyebrows will change as the pigment gradually settles into the skin. Below are the stages of the healing process:

1. **Day 1: Immediately After the Procedure**
   Your eyebrows will look very intense, dark, and prominent. The skin may be slightly swollen and red. The pigment will appear darker than the final result, as the dye is still on the surface of the skin.

2. **Days 2–3**
   Swelling starts to subside, and the skin around the eyebrows may feel dry or tight.
   The eyebrows will still appear dark, but the skin begins to form a light protective layer.

3. **Days 4–7**
   Exfoliation begins. Scabs may form and fall off naturally, so it's important not to touch, scratch, or try to speed up the process.
   Your eyebrows may look uneven or have „empty" spots, but this is a normal part of healing as the pigment settles.

4. **Days 7–14**
   The scabs gradually fall off, and the pigment may look much lighter. Many people feel that their eyebrows are too light at this stage, but the color will continue to stabilize.
   Continue to avoid excessive washing and using cosmetics on the eyebrow area.

5. **Days 14–21**
   The eyebrows will appear lighter and more natural. Some areas may seem lighter than others, but this is part of the process.
   The pigment begins to settle into the skin, and the final color will start to become more visible.

6. **After 4 Weeks**
   By this point, the eyebrows are fully healed. The color will be 20-50% lighter compared to the first few days post-procedure.
   A touch-up session may be needed to fill any pigment gaps or refine the shape.

Date of your touch-up:

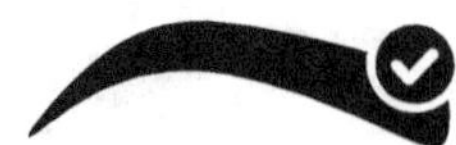

Post-procedure care after micropigmentation

Following a micropigmentation procedure, the skin requires special attention to ensure proper healing and long-lasting, aesthetic results. Below are the recommended post-care instructions:

1. **Hygiene**
   Always wash your hands before touching your eyebrows.
   For the first week, gently cleanse the treated area with lukewarm water.
   Soak a cotton pad in lukewarm water and gently dab your eyebrows, avoiding any rubbing motions.
   Dry the area using a dry cotton pad, again with gentle dabbing to avoid friction.
   Repeat this process 4 times a day at regular intervals.
   For the first two weeks, avoid excessive moisture on the eyebrows (e.g., during baths or showers). After 7-14 days, when the initial healing has occurred, you may begin using a gentle micellar water for cleansing. Avoid products containing alcohol or harsh ingredients.

2. **Preventing Irritation**
   Do not scratch or rub your eyebrows, even if small scabs form. Allow the scabs to fall off naturally to avoid scarring or pigment loss.
   Avoid applying makeup to the eyebrow area until fully healed (approximately 7-14 days).
   For at least 14 days, avoid saunas, swimming pools, hot baths, and excessive sweating, as these can cause the pigment to fade or irritate the skin.

3. **Sun Protection**
   Avoid sun exposure and tanning beds for at least 4 weeks. UV radiation can cause the pigment to fade.
   Once your eyebrows are fully healed, apply a high SPF sunscreen to protect the pigment from fading.

4. **Avoiding Intensive Cosmetic Treatments**
   For 4-6 weeks post-procedure, avoid facial treatments such as chemical peels, laser treatments, or the use of strong creams around the eyebrow area, as these may weaken the pigment.

5. **Consulting a Specialist**
   If you have any concerns or notice unusual symptoms such as excessive redness, swelling, or oozing, contact the cosmetologist who performed the procedure.

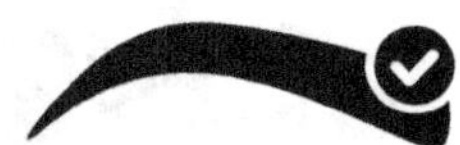

Healing process after micropigmentation

The healing process following permanent eyebrow makeup takes place in several stages and usually lasts between 4 to 6 weeks. During this time, the appearance of your eyebrows will change as the pigment gradually settles into the skin. Below are the stages of the healing process:

1. **Day 1: Immediately After the Procedure**
   Your eyebrows will look very intense, dark, and prominent. The skin may be slightly swollen and red. The pigment will appear darker than the final result, as the dye is still on the surface of the skin.

2. **Days 2–3**
   Swelling starts to subside, and the skin around the eyebrows may feel dry or tight.
   The eyebrows will still appear dark, but the skin begins to form a light protective layer.

3. **Days 4–7**
   Exfoliation begins. Scabs may form and fall off naturally, so it's important not to touch, scratch, or try to speed up the process.
   Your eyebrows may look uneven or have „empty" spots, but this is a normal part of healing as the pigment settles.

4. **Days 7–14**
   The scabs gradually fall off, and the pigment may look much lighter. Many people feel that their eyebrows are too light at this stage, but the color will continue to stabilize.
   Continue to avoid excessive washing and using cosmetics on the eyebrow area.

5. **Days 14–21**
   The eyebrows will appear lighter and more natural. Some areas may seem lighter than others, but this is part of the process.
   The pigment begins to settle into the skin, and the final color will start to become more visible.

6. **After 4 Weeks**
   By this point, the eyebrows are fully healed. The color will be 20-50% lighter compared to the first few days post-procedure.
   A touch-up session may be needed to fill any pigment gaps or refine the shape.

Date of your touch-up:

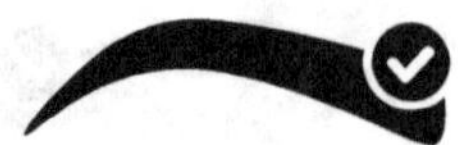

Post-procedure care after micropigmentation

Following a micropigmentation procedure, the skin requires special attention to ensure proper healing and long-lasting, aesthetic results. Below are the recommended post-care instructions:

1. **Hygiene**
   Always wash your hands before touching your eyebrows.
   For the first week, gently cleanse the treated area with lukewarm water.
   Soak a cotton pad in lukewarm water and gently dab your eyebrows, avoiding any rubbing motions.
   Dry the area using a dry cotton pad, again with gentle dabbing to avoid friction.
   Repeat this process 4 times a day at regular intervals.
   For the first two weeks, avoid excessive moisture on the eyebrows (e.g., during baths or showers). After 7-14 days, when the initial healing has occurred, you may begin using a gentle micellar water for cleansing. Avoid products containing alcohol or harsh ingredients.

2. **Preventing Irritation**
   Do not scratch or rub your eyebrows, even if small scabs form. Allow the scabs to fall off naturally to avoid scarring or pigment loss.
   Avoid applying makeup to the eyebrow area until fully healed (approximately 7-14 days).
   For at least 14 days, avoid saunas, swimming pools, hot baths, and excessive sweating, as these can cause the pigment to fade or irritate the skin.

3. **Sun Protection**
   Avoid sun exposure and tanning beds for at least 4 weeks. UV radiation can cause the pigment to fade.
   Once your eyebrows are fully healed, apply a high SPF sunscreen to protect the pigment from fading.

4. **Avoiding Intensive Cosmetic Treatments**
   For 4-6 weeks post-procedure, avoid facial treatments such as chemical peels, laser treatments, or the use of strong creams around the eyebrow area, as these may weaken the pigment.

5. **Consulting a Specialist**
   If you have any concerns or notice unusual symptoms such as excessive redness, swelling, or oozing, contact the cosmetologist who performed the procedure.

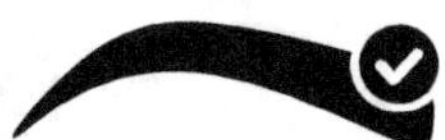

Healing process after micropigmentation

The healing process following permanent eyebrow makeup takes place in several stages and usually lasts between 4 to 6 weeks. During this time, the appearance of your eyebrows will change as the pigment gradually settles into the skin. Below are the stages of the healing process:

① **Day 1: Immediately After the Procedure**
Your eyebrows will look very intense, dark, and prominent. The skin may be slightly swollen and red. The pigment will appear darker than the final result, as the dye is still on the surface of the skin.

② **Days 2–3**
Swelling starts to subside, and the skin around the eyebrows may feel dry or tight.
The eyebrows will still appear dark, but the skin begins to form a light protective layer.

③ **Days 4–7**
Exfoliation begins. Scabs may form and fall off naturally, so it's important not to touch, scratch, or try to speed up the process.
Your eyebrows may look uneven or have „empty" spots, but this is a normal part of healing as the pigment settles.

④ **Days 7–14**
The scabs gradually fall off, and the pigment may look much lighter. Many people feel that their eyebrows are too light at this stage, but the color will continue to stabilize.
Continue to avoid excessive washing and using cosmetics on the eyebrow area.

⑤ **Days 14–21**
The eyebrows will appear lighter and more natural. Some areas may seem lighter than others, but this is part of the process.
The pigment begins to settle into the skin, and the final color will start to become more visible.

⑥ **After 4 Weeks**
By this point, the eyebrows are fully healed. The color will be 20-50% lighter compared to the first few days post-procedure.
A touch-up session may be needed to fill any pigment gaps or refine the shape.

Date of your touch-up:

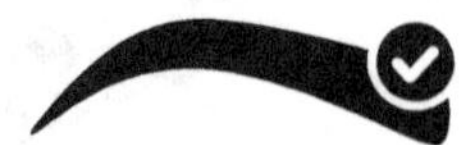

Post-procedure care after micropigmentation

Following a micropigmentation procedure, the skin requires special attention to ensure proper healing and long-lasting, aesthetic results. Below are the recommended post-care instructions:

1. **Hygiene**
   Always wash your hands before touching your eyebrows.
   For the first week, gently cleanse the treated area with lukewarm water.
   Soak a cotton pad in lukewarm water and gently dab your eyebrows, avoiding any rubbing motions.
   Dry the area using a dry cotton pad, again with gentle dabbing to avoid friction.
   Repeat this process 4 times a day at regular intervals.
   For the first two weeks, avoid excessive moisture on the eyebrows (e.g., during baths or showers). After 7-14 days, when the initial healing has occurred, you may begin using a gentle micellar water for cleansing. Avoid products containing alcohol or harsh ingredients.

2. **Preventing Irritation**
   Do not scratch or rub your eyebrows, even if small scabs form. Allow the scabs to fall off naturally to avoid scarring or pigment loss.
   Avoid applying makeup to the eyebrow area until fully healed (approximately 7-14 days).
   For at least 14 days, avoid saunas, swimming pools, hot baths, and excessive sweating, as these can cause the pigment to fade or irritate the skin.

3. **Sun Protection**
   Avoid sun exposure and tanning beds for at least 4 weeks. UV radiation can cause the pigment to fade.
   Once your eyebrows are fully healed, apply a high SPF sunscreen to protect the pigment from fading.

4. **Avoiding Intensive Cosmetic Treatments**
   For 4-6 weeks post-procedure, avoid facial treatments such as chemical peels, laser treatments, or the use of strong creams around the eyebrow area, as these may weaken the pigment.

5. **Consulting a Specialist**
   If you have any concerns or notice unusual symptoms such as excessive redness, swelling, or oozing, contact the cosmetologist who performed the procedure.

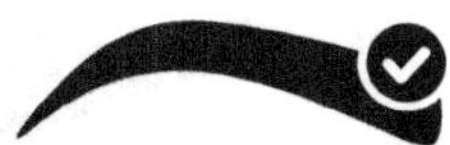

Healing process after micropigmentation

The healing process following permanent eyebrow makeup takes place in several stages and usually lasts between 4 to 6 weeks. During this time, the appearance of your eyebrows will change as the pigment gradually settles into the skin. Below are the stages of the healing process:

1. **Day 1: Immediately After the Procedure**
   Your eyebrows will look very intense, dark, and prominent. The skin may be slightly swollen and red. The pigment will appear darker than the final result, as the dye is still on the surface of the skin.

2. **Days 2–3**
   Swelling starts to subside, and the skin around the eyebrows may feel dry or tight.
   The eyebrows will still appear dark, but the skin begins to form a light protective layer.

3. **Days 4–7**
   Exfoliation begins. Scabs may form and fall off naturally, so it's important not to touch, scratch, or try to speed up the process.
   Your eyebrows may look uneven or have „empty" spots, but this is a normal part of healing as the pigment settles.

4. **Days 7–14**
   The scabs gradually fall off, and the pigment may look much lighter. Many people feel that their eyebrows are too light at this stage, but the color will continue to stabilize.
   Continue to avoid excessive washing and using cosmetics on the eyebrow area.

5. **Days 14–21**
   The eyebrows will appear lighter and more natural. Some areas may seem lighter than others, but this is part of the process.
   The pigment begins to settle into the skin, and the final color will start to become more visible.

6. **After 4 Weeks**
   By this point, the eyebrows are fully healed. The color will be 20-50% lighter compared to the first few days post-procedure.
   A touch-up session may be needed to fill any pigment gaps or refine the shape.

Date of your touch-up:

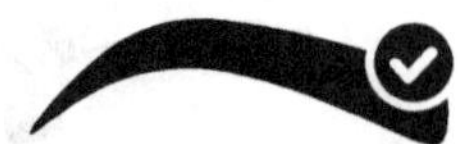

Post-procedure care after micropigmentation

Following a micropigmentation procedure, the skin requires special attention to ensure proper healing and long-lasting, aesthetic results. Below are the recommended post-care instructions:

1. **Hygiene**

   Always wash your hands before touching your eyebrows.

   For the first week, gently cleanse the treated area with lukewarm water.

   Soak a cotton pad in lukewarm water and gently dab your eyebrows, avoiding any rubbing motions.

   Dry the area using a dry cotton pad, again with gentle dabbing to avoid friction.

   Repeat this process 4 times a day at regular intervals.

   For the first two weeks, avoid excessive moisture on the eyebrows (e.g., during baths or showers). After 7-14 days, when the initial healing has occurred, you may begin using a gentle micellar water for cleansing. Avoid products containing alcohol or harsh ingredients.

2. **Preventing Irritation**

   Do not scratch or rub your eyebrows, even if small scabs form. Allow the scabs to fall off naturally to avoid scarring or pigment loss.

   Avoid applying makeup to the eyebrow area until fully healed (approximately 7-14 days).

   For at least 14 days, avoid saunas, swimming pools, hot baths, and excessive sweating, as these can cause the pigment to fade or irritate the skin.

3. **Sun Protection**

   Avoid sun exposure and tanning beds for at least 4 weeks. UV radiation can cause the pigment to fade.

   Once your eyebrows are fully healed, apply a high SPF sunscreen to protect the pigment from fading.

4. **Avoiding Intensive Cosmetic Treatments**

   For 4-6 weeks post-procedure, avoid facial treatments such as chemical peels, laser treatments, or the use of strong creams around the eyebrow area, as these may weaken the pigment.

5. **Consulting a Specialist**

   If you have any concerns or notice unusual symptoms such as excessive redness, swelling, or oozing, contact the cosmetologist who performed the procedure.

Healing process after micropigmentation

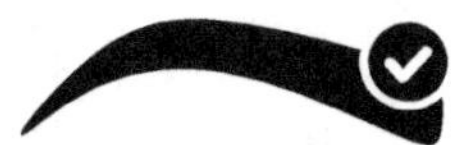

The healing process following permanent eyebrow makeup takes place in several stages and usually lasts between 4 to 6 weeks. During this time, the appearance of your eyebrows will change as the pigment gradually settles into the skin. Below are the stages of the healing process:

1. **Day 1: Immediately After the Procedure**
   Your eyebrows will look very intense, dark, and prominent. The skin may be slightly swollen and red. The pigment will appear darker than the final result, as the dye is still on the surface of the skin.

2. **Days 2–3**
   Swelling starts to subside, and the skin around the eyebrows may feel dry or tight.
   The eyebrows will still appear dark, but the skin begins to form a light protective layer.

3. **Days 4–7**
   Exfoliation begins. Scabs may form and fall off naturally, so it's important not to touch, scratch, or try to speed up the process.
   Your eyebrows may look uneven or have „empty" spots, but this is a normal part of healing as the pigment settles.

4. **Days 7–14**
   The scabs gradually fall off, and the pigment may look much lighter. Many people feel that their eyebrows are too light at this stage, but the color will continue to stabilize.
   Continue to avoid excessive washing and using cosmetics on the eyebrow area.

5. **Days 14–21**
   The eyebrows will appear lighter and more natural. Some areas may seem lighter than others, but this is part of the process.
   The pigment begins to settle into the skin, and the final color will start to become more visible.

6. **After 4 Weeks**
   By this point, the eyebrows are fully healed. The color will be 20-50% lighter compared to the first few days post-procedure.
   A touch-up session may be needed to fill any pigment gaps or refine the shape.

Date of your touch-up:

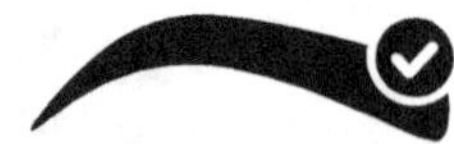

Post-procedure care after micropigmentation

Following a micropigmentation procedure, the skin requires special attention to ensure proper healing and long-lasting, aesthetic results. Below are the recommended post-care instructions:

1. **Hygiene**

   Always wash your hands before touching your eyebrows.

   For the first week, gently cleanse the treated area with lukewarm water.

   Soak a cotton pad in lukewarm water and gently dab your eyebrows, avoiding any rubbing motions.

   Dry the area using a dry cotton pad, again with gentle dabbing to avoid friction.

   Repeat this process 4 times a day at regular intervals.

   For the first two weeks, avoid excessive moisture on the eyebrows (e.g., during baths or showers). After 7-14 days, when the initial healing has occurred, you may begin using a gentle micellar water for cleansing. Avoid products containing alcohol or harsh ingredients.

2. **Preventing Irritation**

   Do not scratch or rub your eyebrows, even if small scabs form. Allow the scabs to fall off naturally to avoid scarring or pigment loss.

   Avoid applying makeup to the eyebrow area until fully healed (approximately 7-14 days).

   For at least 14 days, avoid saunas, swimming pools, hot baths, and excessive sweating, as these can cause the pigment to fade or irritate the skin.

3. **Sun Protection**

   Avoid sun exposure and tanning beds for at least 4 weeks. UV radiation can cause the pigment to fade.

   Once your eyebrows are fully healed, apply a high SPF sunscreen to protect the pigment from fading.

4. **Avoiding Intensive Cosmetic Treatments**

   For 4-6 weeks post-procedure, avoid facial treatments such as chemical peels, laser treatments, or the use of strong creams around the eyebrow area, as these may weaken the pigment.

5. **Consulting a Specialist**

   If you have any concerns or notice unusual symptoms such as excessive redness, swelling, or oozing, contact the cosmetologist who performed the procedure.

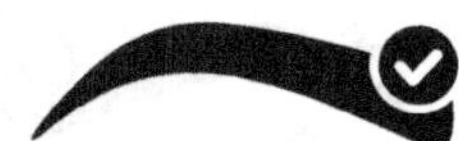

Healing process after micropigmentation

The healing process following permanent eyebrow makeup takes place in several stages and usually lasts between 4 to 6 weeks. During this time, the appearance of your eyebrows will change as the pigment gradually settles into the skin. Below are the stages of the healing process:

1. **Day 1: Immediately After the Procedure**
   Your eyebrows will look very intense, dark, and prominent. The skin may be slightly swollen and red. The pigment will appear darker than the final result, as the dye is still on the surface of the skin.

2. **Days 2–3**
   Swelling starts to subside, and the skin around the eyebrows may feel dry or tight.
   The eyebrows will still appear dark, but the skin begins to form a light protective layer.

3. **Days 4–7**
   Exfoliation begins. Scabs may form and fall off naturally, so it's important not to touch, scratch, or try to speed up the process.
   Your eyebrows may look uneven or have „empty" spots, but this is a normal part of healing as the pigment settles.

4. **Days 7–14**
   The scabs gradually fall off, and the pigment may look much lighter. Many people feel that their eyebrows are too light at this stage, but the color will continue to stabilize.
   Continue to avoid excessive washing and using cosmetics on the eyebrow area.

5. **Days 14–21**
   The eyebrows will appear lighter and more natural. Some areas may seem lighter than others, but this is part of the process.
   The pigment begins to settle into the skin, and the final color will start to become more visible.

6. **After 4 Weeks**
   By this point, the eyebrows are fully healed. The color will be 20-50% lighter compared to the first few days post-procedure.
   A touch-up session may be needed to fill any pigment gaps or refine the shape.

Date of your touch-up:

Post-procedure care after micropigmentation

Following a micropigmentation procedure, the skin requires special attention to ensure proper healing and long-lasting, aesthetic results. Below are the recommended post-care instructions:

1. **Hygiene**

   Always wash your hands before touching your eyebrows.

   For the first week, gently cleanse the treated area with lukewarm water.

   Soak a cotton pad in lukewarm water and gently dab your eyebrows, avoiding any rubbing motions.

   Dry the area using a dry cotton pad, again with gentle dabbing to avoid friction.

   Repeat this process 4 times a day at regular intervals.

   For the first two weeks, avoid excessive moisture on the eyebrows (e.g., during baths or showers). After 7-14 days, when the initial healing has occurred, you may begin using a gentle micellar water for cleansing. Avoid products containing alcohol or harsh ingredients.

2. **Preventing Irritation**

   Do not scratch or rub your eyebrows, even if small scabs form. Allow the scabs to fall off naturally to avoid scarring or pigment loss.

   Avoid applying makeup to the eyebrow area until fully healed (approximately 7-14 days).

   For at least 14 days, avoid saunas, swimming pools, hot baths, and excessive sweating, as these can cause the pigment to fade or irritate the skin.

3. **Sun Protection**

   Avoid sun exposure and tanning beds for at least 4 weeks. UV radiation can cause the pigment to fade.

   Once your eyebrows are fully healed, apply a high SPF sunscreen to protect the pigment from fading.

4. **Avoiding Intensive Cosmetic Treatments**

   For 4-6 weeks post-procedure, avoid facial treatments such as chemical peels, laser treatments, or the use of strong creams around the eyebrow area, as these may weaken the pigment.

5. **Consulting a Specialist**

   If you have any concerns or notice unusual symptoms such as excessive redness, swelling, or oozing, contact the cosmetologist who performed the procedure.

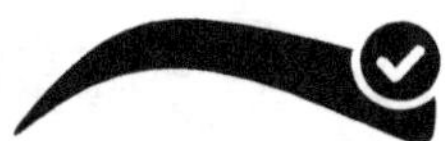

Healing process after micropigmentation

The healing process following permanent eyebrow makeup takes place in several stages and usually lasts between 4 to 6 weeks. During this time, the appearance of your eyebrows will change as the pigment gradually settles into the skin. Below are the stages of the healing process:

1. **Day 1: Immediately After the Procedure**
   Your eyebrows will look very intense, dark, and prominent. The skin may be slightly swollen and red. The pigment will appear darker than the final result, as the dye is still on the surface of the skin.

2. **Days 2–3**
   Swelling starts to subside, and the skin around the eyebrows may feel dry or tight.
   The eyebrows will still appear dark, but the skin begins to form a light protective layer.

3. **Days 4–7**
   Exfoliation begins. Scabs may form and fall off naturally, so it's important not to touch, scratch, or try to speed up the process.
   Your eyebrows may look uneven or have „empty" spots, but this is a normal part of healing as the pigment settles.

4. **Days 7–14**
   The scabs gradually fall off, and the pigment may look much lighter. Many people feel that their eyebrows are too light at this stage, but the color will continue to stabilize.
   Continue to avoid excessive washing and using cosmetics on the eyebrow area.

5. **Days 14–21**
   The eyebrows will appear lighter and more natural. Some areas may seem lighter than others, but this is part of the process.
   The pigment begins to settle into the skin, and the final color will start to become more visible.

6. **After 4 Weeks**
   By this point, the eyebrows are fully healed. The color will be 20-50% lighter compared to the first few days post-procedure.
   A touch-up session may be needed to fill any pigment gaps or refine the shape.

Date of your touch-up:

Post-procedure care after micropigmentation

Following a micropigmentation procedure, the skin requires special attention to ensure proper healing and long-lasting, aesthetic results. Below are the recommended post-care instructions:

1. **Hygiene**
   Always wash your hands before touching your eyebrows.
   For the first week, gently cleanse the treated area with lukewarm water.
   Soak a cotton pad in lukewarm water and gently dab your eyebrows, avoiding any rubbing motions.
   Dry the area using a dry cotton pad, again with gentle dabbing to avoid friction.
   Repeat this process 4 times a day at regular intervals.
   For the first two weeks, avoid excessive moisture on the eyebrows (e.g., during baths or showers). After 7-14 days, when the initial healing has occurred, you may begin using a gentle micellar water for cleansing. Avoid products containing alcohol or harsh ingredients.

2. **Preventing Irritation**
   Do not scratch or rub your eyebrows, even if small scabs form. Allow the scabs to fall off naturally to avoid scarring or pigment loss.
   Avoid applying makeup to the eyebrow area until fully healed (approximately 7-14 days).
   For at least 14 days, avoid saunas, swimming pools, hot baths, and excessive sweating, as these can cause the pigment to fade or irritate the skin.

3. **Sun Protection**
   Avoid sun exposure and tanning beds for at least 4 weeks. UV radiation can cause the pigment to fade.
   Once your eyebrows are fully healed, apply a high SPF sunscreen to protect the pigment from fading.

4. **Avoiding Intensive Cosmetic Treatments**
   For 4-6 weeks post-procedure, avoid facial treatments such as chemical peels, laser treatments, or the use of strong creams around the eyebrow area, as these may weaken the pigment.

5. **Consulting a Specialist**
   If you have any concerns or notice unusual symptoms such as excessive redness, swelling, or oozing, contact the cosmetologist who performed the procedure.

Healing process after micropigmentation

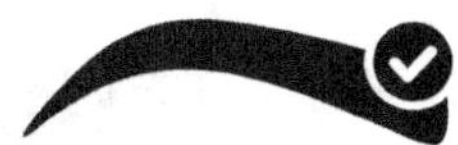

The healing process following permanent eyebrow makeup takes place in several stages and usually lasts between 4 to 6 weeks. During this time, the appearance of your eyebrows will change as the pigment gradually settles into the skin. Below are the stages of the healing process:

1. **Day 1: Immediately After the Procedure**
   Your eyebrows will look very intense, dark, and prominent. The skin may be slightly swollen and red. The pigment will appear darker than the final result, as the dye is still on the surface of the skin.

2. **Days 2–3**
   Swelling starts to subside, and the skin around the eyebrows may feel dry or tight.
   The eyebrows will still appear dark, but the skin begins to form a light protective layer.

3. **Days 4–7**
   Exfoliation begins. Scabs may form and fall off naturally, so it's important not to touch, scratch, or try to speed up the process.
   Your eyebrows may look uneven or have „empty" spots, but this is a normal part of healing as the pigment settles.

4. **Days 7–14**
   The scabs gradually fall off, and the pigment may look much lighter. Many people feel that their eyebrows are too light at this stage, but the color will continue to stabilize.
   Continue to avoid excessive washing and using cosmetics on the eyebrow area.

5. **Days 14–21**
   The eyebrows will appear lighter and more natural. Some areas may seem lighter than others, but this is part of the process.
   The pigment begins to settle into the skin, and the final color will start to become more visible.

6. **After 4 Weeks**
   By this point, the eyebrows are fully healed. The color will be 20-50% lighter compared to the first few days post-procedure.
   A touch-up session may be needed to fill any pigment gaps or refine the shape.

Date of your touch-up:

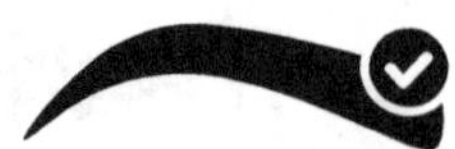

Post-procedure care after micropigmentation

Following a micropigmentation procedure, the skin requires special attention to ensure proper healing and long-lasting, aesthetic results. Below are the recommended post-care instructions:

1. **Hygiene**

   Always wash your hands before touching your eyebrows.

   For the first week, gently cleanse the treated area with lukewarm water.

   Soak a cotton pad in lukewarm water and gently dab your eyebrows, avoiding any rubbing motions.

   Dry the area using a dry cotton pad, again with gentle dabbing to avoid friction.

   Repeat this process 4 times a day at regular intervals.

   For the first two weeks, avoid excessive moisture on the eyebrows (e.g., during baths or showers). After 7-14 days, when the initial healing has occurred, you may begin using a gentle micellar water for cleansing. Avoid products containing alcohol or harsh ingredients.

2. **Preventing Irritation**

   Do not scratch or rub your eyebrows, even if small scabs form. Allow the scabs to fall off naturally to avoid scarring or pigment loss.

   Avoid applying makeup to the eyebrow area until fully healed (approximately 7-14 days).

   For at least 14 days, avoid saunas, swimming pools, hot baths, and excessive sweating, as these can cause the pigment to fade or irritate the skin.

3. **Sun Protection**

   Avoid sun exposure and tanning beds for at least 4 weeks. UV radiation can cause the pigment to fade.

   Once your eyebrows are fully healed, apply a high SPF sunscreen to protect the pigment from fading.

4. **Avoiding Intensive Cosmetic Treatments**

   For 4-6 weeks post-procedure, avoid facial treatments such as chemical peels, laser treatments, or the use of strong creams around the eyebrow area, as these may weaken the pigment.

5. **Consulting a Specialist**

   If you have any concerns or notice unusual symptoms such as excessive redness, swelling, or oozing, contact the cosmetologist who performed the procedure.

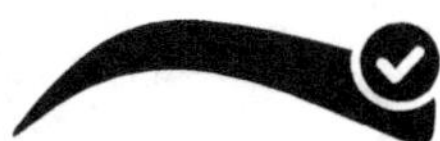

Healing process after micropigmentation

The healing process following permanent eyebrow makeup takes place in several stages and usually lasts between 4 to 6 weeks. During this time, the appearance of your eyebrows will change as the pigment gradually settles into the skin. Below are the stages of the healing process:

1. **Day 1: Immediately After the Procedure**
   Your eyebrows will look very intense, dark, and prominent. The skin may be slightly swollen and red. The pigment will appear darker than the final result, as the dye is still on the surface of the skin.

2. **Days 2–3**
   Swelling starts to subside, and the skin around the eyebrows may feel dry or tight.
   The eyebrows will still appear dark, but the skin begins to form a light protective layer.

3. **Days 4–7**
   Exfoliation begins. Scabs may form and fall off naturally, so it's important not to touch, scratch, or try to speed up the process.
   Your eyebrows may look uneven or have „empty" spots, but this is a normal part of healing as the pigment settles.

4. **Days 7–14**
   The scabs gradually fall off, and the pigment may look much lighter. Many people feel that their eyebrows are too light at this stage, but the color will continue to stabilize.
   Continue to avoid excessive washing and using cosmetics on the eyebrow area.

5. **Days 14–21**
   The eyebrows will appear lighter and more natural. Some areas may seem lighter than others, but this is part of the process.
   The pigment begins to settle into the skin, and the final color will start to become more visible.

6. **After 4 Weeks**
   By this point, the eyebrows are fully healed. The color will be 20-50% lighter compared to the first few days post-procedure.
   A touch-up session may be needed to fill any pigment gaps or refine the shape.

Date of your touch-up:

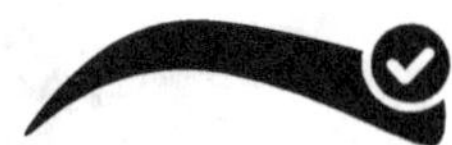

Post-procedure care after micropigmentation

Following a micropigmentation procedure, the skin requires special attention to ensure proper healing and long-lasting, aesthetic results. Below are the recommended post-care instructions:

① **Hygiene**

Always wash your hands before touching your eyebrows.

For the first week, gently cleanse the treated area with lukewarm water.

Soak a cotton pad in lukewarm water and gently dab your eyebrows, avoiding any rubbing motions.

Dry the area using a dry cotton pad, again with gentle dabbing to avoid friction.

Repeat this process 4 times a day at regular intervals.

For the first two weeks, avoid excessive moisture on the eyebrows (e.g., during baths or showers). After 7-14 days, when the initial healing has occurred, you may begin using a gentle micellar water for cleansing. Avoid products containing alcohol or harsh ingredients.

② **Preventing Irritation**

Do not scratch or rub your eyebrows, even if small scabs form. Allow the scabs to fall off naturally to avoid scarring or pigment loss.

Avoid applying makeup to the eyebrow area until fully healed (approximately 7-14 days).

For at least 14 days, avoid saunas, swimming pools, hot baths, and excessive sweating, as these can cause the pigment to fade or irritate the skin.

③ **Sun Protection**

Avoid sun exposure and tanning beds for at least 4 weeks. UV radiation can cause the pigment to fade.

Once your eyebrows are fully healed, apply a high SPF sunscreen to protect the pigment from fading.

④ **Avoiding Intensive Cosmetic Treatments**

For 4-6 weeks post-procedure, avoid facial treatments such as chemical peels, laser treatments, or the use of strong creams around the eyebrow area, as these may weaken the pigment.

⑤ **Consulting a Specialist**

If you have any concerns or notice unusual symptoms such as excessive redness, swelling, or oozing, contact the cosmetologist who performed the procedure.

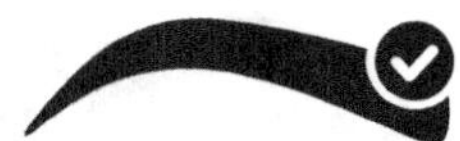

Healing process after micropigmentation

The healing process following permanent eyebrow makeup takes place in several stages and usually lasts between 4 to 6 weeks. During this time, the appearance of your eyebrows will change as the pigment gradually settles into the skin. Below are the stages of the healing process:

1. **Day 1: Immediately After the Procedure**
   Your eyebrows will look very intense, dark, and prominent. The skin may be slightly swollen and red. The pigment will appear darker than the final result, as the dye is still on the surface of the skin.

2. **Days 2–3**
   Swelling starts to subside, and the skin around the eyebrows may feel dry or tight.
   The eyebrows will still appear dark, but the skin begins to form a light protective layer.

3. **Days 4–7**
   Exfoliation begins. Scabs may form and fall off naturally, so it's important not to touch, scratch, or try to speed up the process.
   Your eyebrows may look uneven or have „empty" spots, but this is a normal part of healing as the pigment settles.

4. **Days 7–14**
   The scabs gradually fall off, and the pigment may look much lighter. Many people feel that their eyebrows are too light at this stage, but the color will continue to stabilize.
   Continue to avoid excessive washing and using cosmetics on the eyebrow area.

5. **Days 14–21**
   The eyebrows will appear lighter and more natural. Some areas may seem lighter than others, but this is part of the process.
   The pigment begins to settle into the skin, and the final color will start to become more visible.

6. **After 4 Weeks**
   By this point, the eyebrows are fully healed. The color will be 20-50% lighter compared to the first few days post-procedure.
   A touch-up session may be needed to fill any pigment gaps or refine the shape.

Date of your touch-up:

Post-procedure care after micropigmentation

Following a micropigmentation procedure, the skin requires special attention to ensure proper healing and long-lasting, aesthetic results. Below are the recommended post-care instructions:

1. **Hygiene**
   Always wash your hands before touching your eyebrows.
   For the first week, gently cleanse the treated area with lukewarm water.
   Soak a cotton pad in lukewarm water and gently dab your eyebrows, avoiding any rubbing motions.
   Dry the area using a dry cotton pad, again with gentle dabbing to avoid friction.
   Repeat this process 4 times a day at regular intervals.
   For the first two weeks, avoid excessive moisture on the eyebrows (e.g., during baths or showers). After 7-14 days, when the initial healing has occurred, you may begin using a gentle micellar water for cleansing. Avoid products containing alcohol or harsh ingredients.

2. **Preventing Irritation**
   Do not scratch or rub your eyebrows, even if small scabs form. Allow the scabs to fall off naturally to avoid scarring or pigment loss.
   Avoid applying makeup to the eyebrow area until fully healed (approximately 7-14 days).
   For at least 14 days, avoid saunas, swimming pools, hot baths, and excessive sweating, as these can cause the pigment to fade or irritate the skin.

3. **Sun Protection**
   Avoid sun exposure and tanning beds for at least 4 weeks. UV radiation can cause the pigment to fade.
   Once your eyebrows are fully healed, apply a high SPF sunscreen to protect the pigment from fading.

4. **Avoiding Intensive Cosmetic Treatments**
   For 4-6 weeks post-procedure, avoid facial treatments such as chemical peels, laser treatments, or the use of strong creams around the eyebrow area, as these may weaken the pigment.

5. **Consulting a Specialist**
   If you have any concerns or notice unusual symptoms such as excessive redness, swelling, or oozing, contact the cosmetologist who performed the procedure.

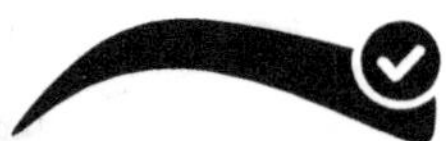

Healing process after micropigmentation

The healing process following permanent eyebrow makeup takes place in several stages and usually lasts between 4 to 6 weeks. During this time, the appearance of your eyebrows will change as the pigment gradually settles into the skin. Below are the stages of the healing process:

1. **Day 1: Immediately After the Procedure**
   Your eyebrows will look very intense, dark, and prominent. The skin may be slightly swollen and red. The pigment will appear darker than the final result, as the dye is still on the surface of the skin.

2. **Days 2–3**
   Swelling starts to subside, and the skin around the eyebrows may feel dry or tight.
   The eyebrows will still appear dark, but the skin begins to form a light protective layer.

3. **Days 4–7**
   Exfoliation begins. Scabs may form and fall off naturally, so it's important not to touch, scratch, or try to speed up the process.
   Your eyebrows may look uneven or have „empty" spots, but this is a normal part of healing as the pigment settles.

4. **Days 7–14**
   The scabs gradually fall off, and the pigment may look much lighter. Many people feel that their eyebrows are too light at this stage, but the color will continue to stabilize.
   Continue to avoid excessive washing and using cosmetics on the eyebrow area.

5. **Days 14–21**
   The eyebrows will appear lighter and more natural. Some areas may seem lighter than others, but this is part of the process.
   The pigment begins to settle into the skin, and the final color will start to become more visible.

6. **After 4 Weeks**
   By this point, the eyebrows are fully healed. The color will be 20-50% lighter compared to the first few days post-procedure.
   A touch-up session may be needed to fill any pigment gaps or refine the shape.

Date of your touch-up:

Post-procedure care after micropigmentation

Following a micropigmentation procedure, the skin requires special attention to ensure proper healing and long-lasting, aesthetic results. Below are the recommended post-care instructions:

1. **Hygiene**

   Always wash your hands before touching your eyebrows.

   For the first week, gently cleanse the treated area with lukewarm water.

   Soak a cotton pad in lukewarm water and gently dab your eyebrows, avoiding any rubbing motions.

   Dry the area using a dry cotton pad, again with gentle dabbing to avoid friction.

   Repeat this process 4 times a day at regular intervals.

   For the first two weeks, avoid excessive moisture on the eyebrows (e.g., during baths or showers). After 7-14 days, when the initial healing has occurred, you may begin using a gentle micellar water for cleansing. Avoid products containing alcohol or harsh ingredients.

2. **Preventing Irritation**

   Do not scratch or rub your eyebrows, even if small scabs form. Allow the scabs to fall off naturally to avoid scarring or pigment loss.

   Avoid applying makeup to the eyebrow area until fully healed (approximately 7-14 days).

   For at least 14 days, avoid saunas, swimming pools, hot baths, and excessive sweating, as these can cause the pigment to fade or irritate the skin.

3. **Sun Protection**

   Avoid sun exposure and tanning beds for at least 4 weeks. UV radiation can cause the pigment to fade.

   Once your eyebrows are fully healed, apply a high SPF sunscreen to protect the pigment from fading.

4. **Avoiding Intensive Cosmetic Treatments**

   For 4-6 weeks post-procedure, avoid facial treatments such as chemical peels, laser treatments, or the use of strong creams around the eyebrow area, as these may weaken the pigment.

5. **Consulting a Specialist**

   If you have any concerns or notice unusual symptoms such as excessive redness, swelling, or oozing, contact the cosmetologist who performed the procedure.

Healing process after micropigmentation

The healing process following permanent eyebrow makeup takes place in several stages and usually lasts between 4 to 6 weeks. During this time, the appearance of your eyebrows will change as the pigment gradually settles into the skin. Below are the stages of the healing process:

1. **Day 1: Immediately After the Procedure**
   Your eyebrows will look very intense, dark, and prominent. The skin may be slightly swollen and red. The pigment will appear darker than the final result, as the dye is still on the surface of the skin.

2. **Days 2–3**
   Swelling starts to subside, and the skin around the eyebrows may feel dry or tight.
   The eyebrows will still appear dark, but the skin begins to form a light protective layer.

3. **Days 4–7**
   Exfoliation begins. Scabs may form and fall off naturally, so it's important not to touch, scratch, or try to speed up the process.
   Your eyebrows may look uneven or have „empty" spots, but this is a normal part of healing as the pigment settles.

4. **Days 7–14**
   The scabs gradually fall off, and the pigment may look much lighter. Many people feel that their eyebrows are too light at this stage, but the color will continue to stabilize.
   Continue to avoid excessive washing and using cosmetics on the eyebrow area.

5. **Days 14–21**
   The eyebrows will appear lighter and more natural. Some areas may seem lighter than others, but this is part of the process.
   The pigment begins to settle into the skin, and the final color will start to become more visible.

6. **After 4 Weeks**
   By this point, the eyebrows are fully healed. The color will be 20-50% lighter compared to the first few days post-procedure.
   A touch-up session may be needed to fill any pigment gaps or refine the shape.

Date of your touch-up:

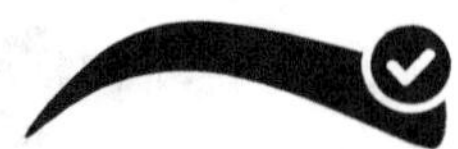

Post-procedure care after micropigmentation

Following a micropigmentation procedure, the skin requires special attention to ensure proper healing and long-lasting, aesthetic results. Below are the recommended post-care instructions:

1. **Hygiene**
   Always wash your hands before touching your eyebrows.
   For the first week, gently cleanse the treated area with lukewarm water.
   Soak a cotton pad in lukewarm water and gently dab your eyebrows, avoiding any rubbing motions.
   Dry the area using a dry cotton pad, again with gentle dabbing to avoid friction.
   Repeat this process 4 times a day at regular intervals.
   For the first two weeks, avoid excessive moisture on the eyebrows (e.g., during baths or showers). After 7-14 days, when the initial healing has occurred, you may begin using a gentle micellar water for cleansing. Avoid products containing alcohol or harsh ingredients.

2. **Preventing Irritation**
   Do not scratch or rub your eyebrows, even if small scabs form. Allow the scabs to fall off naturally to avoid scarring or pigment loss.
   Avoid applying makeup to the eyebrow area until fully healed (approximately 7-14 days).
   For at least 14 days, avoid saunas, swimming pools, hot baths, and excessive sweating, as these can cause the pigment to fade or irritate the skin.

3. **Sun Protection**
   Avoid sun exposure and tanning beds for at least 4 weeks. UV radiation can cause the pigment to fade.
   Once your eyebrows are fully healed, apply a high SPF sunscreen to protect the pigment from fading.

4. **Avoiding Intensive Cosmetic Treatments**
   For 4-6 weeks post-procedure, avoid facial treatments such as chemical peels, laser treatments, or the use of strong creams around the eyebrow area, as these may weaken the pigment.

5. **Consulting a Specialist**
   If you have any concerns or notice unusual symptoms such as excessive redness, swelling, or oozing, contact the cosmetologist who performed the procedure.